Sickle Cell Anemia and Other Hemoglobinopathies

ACADEMIC PRESS RAPID MANUSCRIPT REPRODUCTION

Proceedings of a Symposium on Sickle Cell Anemia, held at the State University of New York, Downstate Medical Center, Brooklyn, New York, and sponsored by the Comprehensive Sickle Cell Anemia Center, March 13th , 1974.

Sickle Cell Anemia and Other Hemoglobinopathies

Edited by

Richard D. Levere

Department of Medicine
State University of New York
College of Medicine
Brooklyn, New York

ACADEMIC PRESS INC., New York San Francisco London 1975

A Subsidiary of Harcourt Brace Jovanovich, Publishers

ACADEMIC PRESS, INC.
111 Fifth Avenue, New York, New York 10003

United Kingdom Edition published by
ACADEMIC PRESS, INC. (LONDON) LTD.
24/28 Oval Road, London NW1

Library of Congress Cataloging in Publication Data

Symposium on Sickle Cell Anemia, New York, 1974
Sickle cell anemia and other hemoglobinopathies.

"Proceedings of a Symposium on Sickle Cell Anemia, held at the State University of New York, Downstate Medical Center, Brooklyn, New York, and sponsored by the Comprehensive Sickle Cell Anemia Center, March 13th, 1974."

1. Sickle cell anemia–Congresses. 2. Hemoglobinopathy–Congresses. I. Levere, Richard D. II. New York (State), Downstate Medical Center, New York. Comprehensive Sickle Cell Anemia Center. III. Title.
[DNLM: 1. Anemia, Sickle cell–Congresses. 2. Hemoglobinopathies–Congresses. WH170 S988s 1974]
RC641.S5S95 (1964) 616.1'51 74-27519
ISBN 0–12–444750–3

PRINTED IN THE UNITED STATES OF AMERICA

CONTENTS

PARTICIPANTS

John F. Bertles, M.D., Department of Medicine, Columbia University, College of Physicians and Surgeons, and Hematology Section, St. Luke's Hospital Center, Amsterdam Avenue at 114th Street, New York, New York 10025.

Robert M. Bookchin, M.D., Department of Medicine, Albert Einstein School of Medicine, 1300 Morris Park Avenue, Bronx, New York 10461.

Dorothy M. Holden, M.D., Department of Medicine, Comprehensive Sickle Cell Anemia Center, Downstate Medical Center, Brooklyn, New York 11203.

Robert F. Murray, Jr., M.D., Departments of Pediatrics and Medicine, and Medical Genetics Unit, Howard University School of Medicine, Box #101, Washington, D.C. 20001.

Ronald L. Nagel, M.D., Department of Medicine, Albert Einstein School of Medicine, 1300 Morris Park Avenue, Bronx, New York 10461.

Ronald F. Rieder, M.D., Department of Medicine, Downstate Medical Center, Brooklyn, New York 11203.

Margaret G. Robinson, M.D., Department of Pediatrics, Downstate Medical Center, Brooklyn, New York 11203.*

Donald L. Rucknagel, Ph.D., Department of Medicine, Howard University College of Medicine, Center for Sickle Cell Anemia, Washington, D.C. 20001 and Department of Human Genetics, University of Michigan, 1133 East Catherine Street, Ann Arbor, Michigan 48104.

*Present Address: Medical College of Ohio at Toledo, Toledo Ohio 43614.

PREFACE

A great deal of information concerning the cellular and subcellular aspects of the synthesis of normal and abnormal hemoglobins has been obtained over the past two decades. Although it is obvious that much more needs to be learned at these basic levels, there is an even greater void in our knowledge of the clinical relationships to already delimited molecular abnormalities as well as of the history of sickle cell anemia and trait. This volume presents the proceedings of a symposium held at the Downstate Medical Center with the goal of bringing to the practicing physician the latest information concerning the molecular basis of the hemoglobinopathies. In addition, this basic material is also discussed in relationship to the pathophysiology of these disorders and current problems of management and therapy are also viewed in this light.

I am indebted to the many members of the faculty and staff of the Downstate Medical Center and the Comprehensive Sickle Cell Anemia Center without whose assistance it would have been impossible to organize and successfully compile the symposium in this volume. In particular, I would like to cite the following for their invaluable aid:

Dorothy M. Holden, M.D.
Bertha M. Kearney
June Lorber
Cecile Nathanson
Charles M. Plotz, M.D.
Mary Walsh
William Wheeler

The Symposium was supported by Grant No. HL 15170 from the N.I.H. Heart and Lung Institute to the Comprehensive Sickle Cell Anemia Center.

THE BIOCHEMICAL GENETICS OF SICKLE CELL ANEMIA AND RELATED HEMOGLOBINOPATHIES

Donald L. Rucknagel, M.D., Ph.D.

Sickle Cell Anemia is an important disease in this country, partly because of the high morbidity that affected persons may experience, and partly, because approximately one out of ten Black people have Sickle Cell Trait. The precise figure is closer to 8% and that's reasonably high as genetic traits go. In approximately one in 150 matings between Negroes both partners have Sickle Cell Trait and in such cases the odds are 25% that each child will have Sickle Cell Anemia, 50% that each will have Sickle Cell Trait and 25% that each child will be normal (Fig. 1). About 1 out of every 600 Black children at birth should have Sickle Cell Anemia. The incidence hasn't been accurately measured, however, nor is the population frequency of Sickle Cell Anemia accurately known, which is another way of saying that we are not really sure of the mortality rate or average longevity of persons with Sickle Cell Anemia.

THE HEMOGLOBIN ELECTROPHORETIC ABNORMALITY

It is relatively easy to diagnose Sickle Cell Anemia. The routine blood count and reticulocyte count are necessary in the differential diagnosis, as we shall see later, but the most specific tool is zone electrophoresis. The hemoglobin is placed on some sort of supporting medium at alkaline pH, such as filter paper, starch gel, a polyacrylamide gel or a cellulose acetate membrane, and an electric current passed through the medium. The pattern in Figure 2 is obtained by applying the hemoglobin to a mylar-backed piece of cellulose acetate.

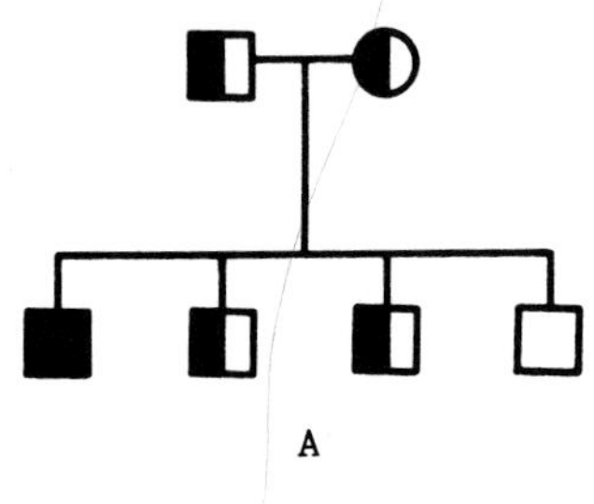

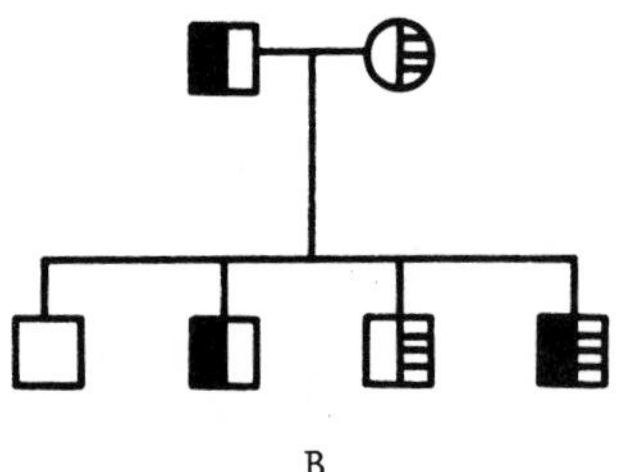

Fig. 1. Pedigrees showing the mode of inheritance of Sickle Cell Anemia (A) *and Sickle Cell* Hb C *Disease* (B)

The open symbol denotes a Hb_{β}^{A} *gene, the solid,* Hb_{β}^{S} *and the cross hatched* Hb_{β}^{C}.

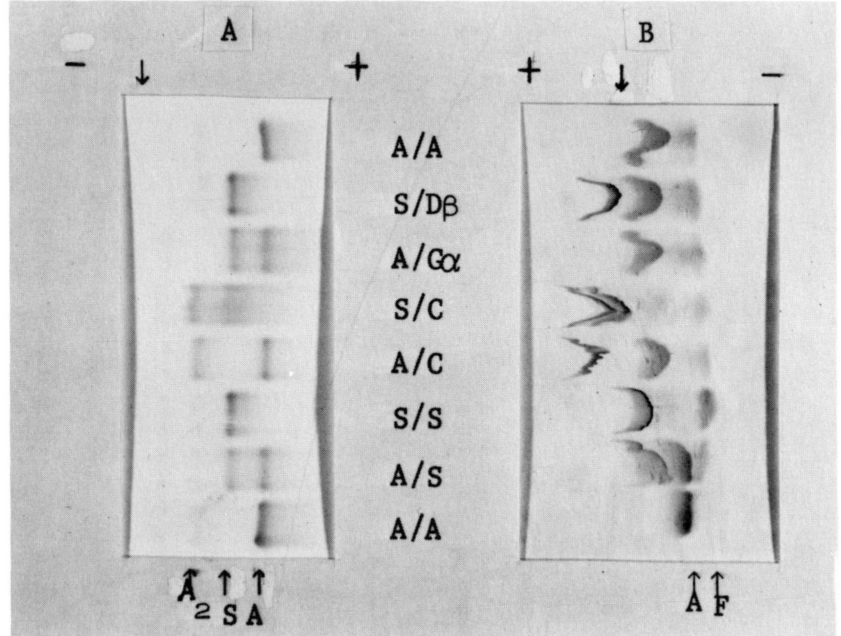

Fig. 2. Electrophoresis of hemoglobin solutions employing two techniques.

A. *Cellulose acetate electrophoresis at* jH 8.6 *stained with ponceav-S. The downward pointing arrow denotes the point of application.* Hb F *migrates between* Hb A *and* Hb S. *The minor band migrating near the origin is carbonic anhydrase enzyme.* Hb C *migrates with the same mobility as* Hb A_2.

B. *Cellulose acetate membrane impregnated with agar in citrate buffer,* pH 6.4 (19). *By this method* Hb F *migrates faster than* Hb A, Hb S *more slowly and* Hb C *even more slowly. Since the relative mobilities are greatly influenced by the amounts of each component present each specimen interpreted on the basis of the number of major components present rather than the position of the various components.*

This is the least expensive and most convenient system today for electrophoresis. Its very high resolution has greatly improved the accuracy of diagnosis. Normal hemoglobin (HbA) migrates more rapidly than that in Sickle Cell Anemia. In Sickle Trait, the blood contains approximately 65% of HbA and 35 to 40 percent of the sickle hemoglobin (HbS). The correlation between the electrophoretic pattern of Figure 2A and the genetic relationship (Fig. 1A), historically speaking, set the stage for the biological revolution that has been underway for the last few decades in that it told us that not only is Sickle Cell Anemia inherited, but also that genes have something to do with protein structure.

It had been recognized in the 1940's that some patients with Sickle Cell Anemia were more mildly affected than others. Instead of having the customary 7 to 8 grams of hemoglobin per 100 ml of blood, some patients have 9 to 11 grams of hemoglobin and instead of having 2 to 4 severe episodes of pain per year, some have so-called crises every 2 to 4 years. I, incidentally, try to avoid the use of the word crisis before patients because it is an emotionally laden term that conjures up inaccurate expectations. I prefer to speak merely about episodes or spells of pain to patients. On the other hand, the word crisis is well entrenched in our terminology and I doubt that we can eliminate its use. Any event in Dr. Neel's [1] genetic studies of Sickle Cell Anemia, published in 1949, he had ascertained 74 families having children with Sickle Cell Anemia. Among them were 2 of these children with mild disease. In both, only one parent had the Sickle Cell Trait. He recognized that these were exceptions to the general rule and of some special significance. Later that year when Pauling, et al.[2] showed the electrophoretic abnormality of hemoglobin S, Dr. Neel, then sent hemoglobin from one of these families to Dr. Itano for electrophoresis. This, then, resulted in the first report of Sickle Cell Hemoglobin C Disease. [3] In this condition, approximately half of the hemoglobin has the mobility of HbS (Fig. 2A) and approximately half of it migrates still more slowly than HbS and is referred to as Hemoglobin C. Figure 2 also shows the electrophoretic pattern of HbC trait (A/C) in which the amount of Hb A exceeds that of Hb C. A mating of a person with Hb C trait with a spouse having Hb S trait produces offspring with Sickle Cell Trait, Hb C trait, Sickle Cell-Hb C Disease and only normal hemoglobin with equal probability (Fig. 1B). Shortly after the discovery of Hb C a group of geneticists and hematologists met and devised a terminology for abnormal hemoglobins. They reserved certain alphabets for various hemoglobins: A (for normal adult hemoglobin), S (for sickle), F (for fetal), and M (for methemoglobin). They skipped the letter "B" because it had already been referred to as the gene for Sickle Cell Anemia. Subsequently described hemoglobins were to be designated alphabetically in order of their discovery; thus, HbC then D, E, G, H, I, etc. Then it became clear that the alphabet would be exceeded, and moreover, the pace of discovery was such that different hemoglobins were getting the same alphabetical designation. A geographic designation was then adopted and, new hemoglobins were provisionally designated with the geographic name...a proprietary name, if you will. As you are well aware, there is a hemoglobin "Flatbush" and a "Riverdale-Bronx", and, there are also Hb's Michigan, Ann Arbor, Wayne, Inkster and Ypsilanti Hemoglobin S.

THE BIOCHEMICAL GENETICS OF HEMOGLOBIN

The hemoglobin A molecule is a tetramer composed of two dissimilar chains. Symbolically it is designated as $\alpha_2\beta_2$. Each chain is composed of approximately 140 residues of the twenty different amino acids found in animal proteins. These amino acid residues are arranged in a specific sequence. The abnormal electrophoretic mobility of Hb S is due to the fact that the Hb S molecule is more electropositive than is Hb A, thus, migrating more slowly toward the positive pole of the electric field. This charge abnormality cannotes an abnormal amino acid composition of Hb S. By the technique of finger-printing or peptide mapping [4], it has been shown that Hb S differs from Hb A by a single amino acid substitution in the beta polypeptide chains. At the sixth position of the amino terminal end the glutamic acid residue normally present is substituted by the amino acid valine. This substitution not only alters the ionic charge of the entire molecule, but it allows gelling of deoxygenated hemoglobin by a process that is still poorly understood but is under intense scrutiny. Hb C differs from Hb A and Hb S in that the very same residue of the beta chain is substituted by lysine, a basic amino acid (Fig. 3).

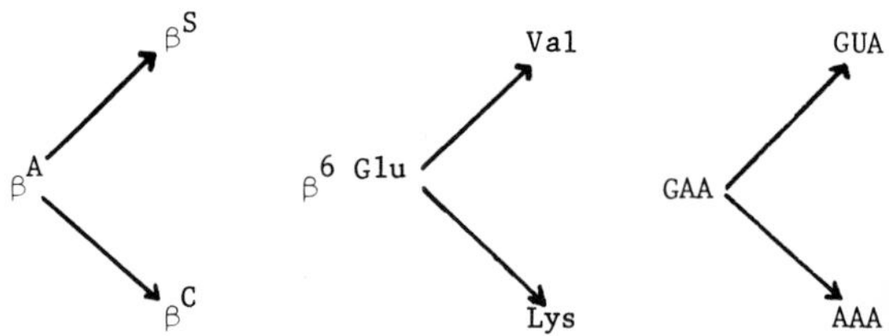

Fig. 3. The relationship between the amino acid substitution and base substitutions in the codons for the β-6 *position is messenger* RNA.

Thus Hb C is even more positively charged than Hb S and therefore migrates more slowly at pH 8.6. These abnormalities are due to abnormalities or mutational events within the DNA which comprises the hemoglobin genes.

DNA is an enormous macromolecule in which four possible purine-pyrimidine base pairs constitute a triplet code such that each three base pairs are equivalent to an amino acid in the polypeptide chains of hemoglobin. That is to say that a hemoglobin structure gene is the proper number of triplets required to encode the sequence of amino acids in the alpha or the beta polypeptide chains. Each gene is transcribed via a single stranded messenger RNA molecule (mRNA) in the nucleus. The mRNA then leaves the nucleus, entering the cytoplasm where it then serves as a template, in conjunction with ribosomes, whereby amino acids are sequentially assembled into polypeptide chains. The base sequence of mRNA is complementary to the base sequence of one of the strands of DNA. Thus, each three bases in the single stranded mRNA molecule are equivalent to an amino acid residue in the hemoglobin polypeptide chain translated from the messenger. The amino acid substitutions in hemoglobins S and C are due to abnormalities in the DNA and mRNA triplet codons equivalent to the sixth amino acid residue. The genetic code, expressed as the mRNA equivalents, has been deciphered through studies in bacteria. It has been shown that GAA is one of the codons equivalent to glutamic acid. In the case of Hb S, a simple error in meiosis causing a base pair substitution in the DNA, in turn changing that GAA to a GUA in mRNA is then responsible for the amino acid substitution, from glutamic to valine (Fig. 3). Likewise, changing that GAA to a AAA is responsible for the glutamic to lysine substitution of Hb S. Both substitutions are possible as a result of single substitutions in the same codon.

Approximately 200 different hemoglobin mutants have been detected in man, most of which differ from Hb A by single amino acid substitutions [5]. If we compare the amino acid substitutions of all of those mutant hemoglobins with the genetic code as deciphered in bacteria the vast majority of the unknown hemoglobins are consistant with single base substitutions in the triplet codon assignments derived from bacterial systems. In other words, the genetic code from bacteria to man is universal, and the large number of mutants of hemoglobin has provided a test of the universality of the code.

Approximately 25 mutants migrate like Hb S; these are generically designated D or G hemoglobins. Although the variants shown in Fig. 2 migrate more slowly than hemoglobin A, the amino acid substitution can also result in a molecule that is more electro-negative and, therefore, at alkaline pH migrates more rapidly than hemoglobin A. Those that migrate faster than A, with a minus 2 net charge, are referred to as J hemoglobins, whereas those that migrate with a minus 4 charge are designated either N or I, the latter migrating slightly faster. Thus, Hb I migrates as far ahead of Hb A as Hb C does behind Hb A. Approximately half of the substitutions affect either the alpha or the beta chains. A growing number of mutants are also being found in the gamma and delta chains of Hb F and Hb A, respectively (Reviewed in reference [5]). The genes that determine the amino acid sequence of the alpha and beta chains, the $\underline{Hb_{\alpha}}$ and $\underline{Hb_{\beta}}$ structural genes, are not closely linke That is to say, they are either on different chromosome or they are so far apart on the same chromosome that crossing-over occurs 50% of the time.

Heterozygotes for the $\underline{Hb_{\alpha}}$ mutants possess only 15 to 20 percent of abnormal hemoglobin, whereas beta chai variants are characterized by 40 percent of the abnormal component. This is most likely due to the presence of two $\underline{Hb_{\alpha}}$ loci [6,7]. Therefore a variant chain is diluted by the α^{A} chains produced by the remaining three $\underline{Hb}^{A}$ alleles. Heterogeneity in the amount of HbGα-Philadelphia might be due to the presence of chromosome with one or two $\underline{Hb_{\alpha}}$ loci in the American negro genome [8]

A number of minor hemoglobins also manifest geneti variation. Thus, HbA_2 ($\alpha_2\delta_2$) , comprise 2 percent of the total hemoglobin. Approximately 2 percent of Ameri can negroes are carriers for a delta chain mutant, HbB_2.

Fetal hemoglobin ($\alpha_2\gamma_2$) comprises 75% of the hemoglobin at birth falling to the adult levels of 1 to 2% by 9 months of age. Hb F is elevated to 10 to 20% of the total hemoglobin in approximately half of the patients with Sickle Cell Anemia. It is also greatly elevated in thalassemia major and less so in thalassemia trait. The genetics of hemoglobin has become considerably more complex in the past few years with the realization that there are at least two and perhaps four gamma chain structural loci [10,11]. The genes for the beta, gamma and delta chains are closely linked [12,13].

SCREENING FOR ABNORMAL HEMOGLOBINS

The simplest technique for detecting sickling is the solubility test, first marketed by the Ortho Company under the proprietary name Sickledex. Since then numerous modifications have been marked, all using the same principle. Many of these have been compared, some work well, others do not [14]. The principle of the solubility test is that deoxygenated HbS is 1/50th as soluble as HbA. The reagent is a combination of saponin; a hemolyzing agent, 2.5 molar phosphate; which salts out the HbS, and dithionite; which deoxygenates the solution. The test is performed simply by adding 0.02 ml of whole blood to 2 ml of reagent. If the tube is clear after approximately 10 to 15 minutes, HbS is not present. If the tube is too turbed to read printed material through it, HbS is present. The advantages of the test are the simplicity, the speed, the economy, and the fact that trained personnel are not required. When proprietary tests are employed the cost per test is 35 cents to approximately one dollar per test, exclusive of technician time. Several recipes have been published, however, which reduce the cost to pennies per test. The major disadvantage with the solubility test is that, given a positive test, one cannot be certain whether the genotype is A/S, S/S, S/C, or other combination with HbS. In many community screening programs employing only this technique the subjects with a positive test must then be referred at considerable expense, loss of work, and generation of anxiety. False negative results are possible if the subject tested is anemic, and false positives result from hyperlipidemia, macro and hypergammaglobulinemia. The test also fails to detect HbC trait or many other abnormal hemoglobins that might be relevant in the genetic counseling context. I shall return to the solubility test, but at the moment, let me emphasize that for all of these reasons an electrophoretic method should be part of every screening program.

The electrophoretic pattern in Figure 1 are relatively expensive and require anti-coagulated venous blood. To centrifuge the blood, remove the plasma, wash the cells, lyse the cells by adding water, and extract the cell membrane and lipids with high speed centrifugation and electrophorese costs approximately five to ten dollars per specimen. To detect variation in the major components it is much more rapid and inexpensive to apply whole blood directly to the electrophoretic medium. Figure 4 is made on a 2 3/4 x 3 inch plate of cellulose acetate.

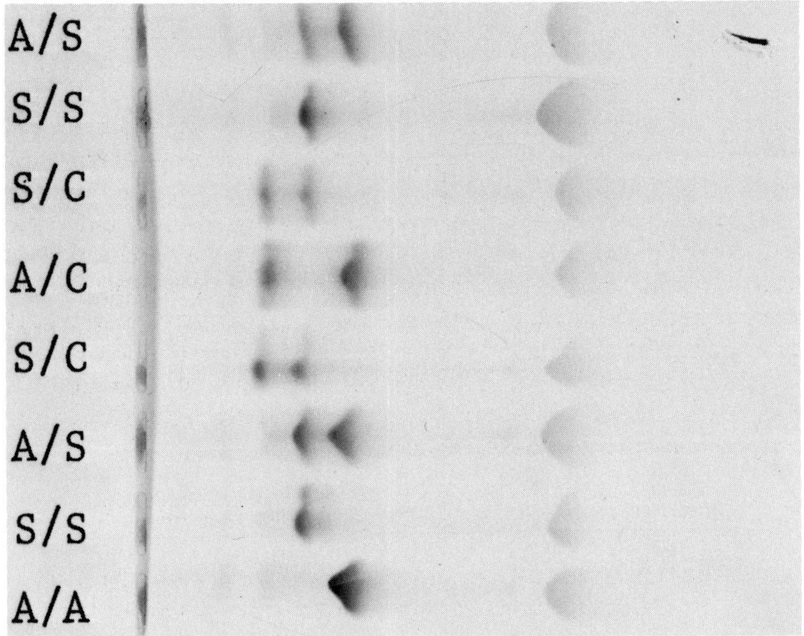

Fig. 4. Screening electrophoresis performed by applying whole blood to the cellulose acetate membrane. The component with the fastest mobility is serum albumin.

A small drop of water or 2 percent KCN, neutralized with acetic acid, is placed in the wells of the applicator along with a small drop of blood. The pattern is stained with Ponceau-S although the hemoglobin is clearly visible without staining. Serum albumin migrates ahead of the hemoglobin and may migrate off the plate. Occasionally serum beta globulin is located near the HbA band; in such patterns the procedure should be repeated and the pattern inspected prior to staining. If the abnormal band is absent but reappears upon staining it is probably a serum protein. If doubt still remains, wash the cells before preparing the hemolysate. Employing the whole blood technique one can differentiate Sickle Cell Trait, Sickle Hemoglobin C, Sickle Cell Anemia, or Hb C Trait from normal in only 15 to 30 minutes. It is therefore possible to admit a patient, prick his or her finger, and while the laboratory work is in progress, educate the patient with audio-visual aids. The subject's understanding can then be assessed and the counseling performed when the laboratory results are completed. Both the screening and counseling can therefore be performed in one visit at minimum expense and inconvenience to the subject. With this method, Dr. Charles Whitten in Detroit screens and counsels "on-the-spot" 30,000 people per year with both a mobile bus and a permanent facility. If only electrophoresis is employed a small proportion of subjects with the electrophoretic pattern of Sickle Cell Trait will, in fact, be heterozygotes for the HbD or HbG. Therefore, it is advisable to include the solubility test along with electrophoresis.

PHENOTYPES SIMILAR TO SICKLE CELL ANEMIA

The electrophoretic pattern of Sickle Cell Anemia can be readily recognized. Laboratories frequently notify physicians that a given specimen contains SS hemoglobin. That statement implies that the subject has two $\underline{Hb}_{\beta}^{S}$ genes, and it is an intellectual trap for the physician because there are three other genotypes, in which the subject has only one $\underline{Hb_{\beta}}^{S}$ gene plus another mutant gene that give the same pattern. I suggest that unless the laboratory has evaluated all of the hematologic data, it may be preferable for the laboratory report to simply describe the electrophoretic pattern, e.g., "mostly HbS present",or that the statement read "compatible with Sickle Cell Anemia".

SICKLE CELL HEMOGLOBIN D SYNDROMES

There are about twenty-five (25) other hemoglobins in which a single amino acid substitution in either the alpha or the beta chain alters the charge of the molecule in a fashion similar to that of sickle hemoglobin [15]. These hemoglobins migrate like S but do not sickle. As noted above, these are referred to as either D or G hemoglobins. If a person inherits a D hemoglobin gene from one parent and a $\underline{Hb_\beta}^S$ from the other, that person has no normal hemoglobin and apparently has only sickle hemoglobin on the electrophoretic pattern (Fig. 2A) if that substitution is on the beta chain. The component with the mobility of HbS is, in fact, a mixture of the two abnormal hemoglobins. If the HbG substitution is on the alpha chain the electrophoretic pattern may be more complex [16]. Thus, a person heterozygous for the $\underline{Hb_\alpha}^G$ and $\underline{Hb_\beta}^S$ has three components with the mobilities of HbA, S, and HbC. The component with the mobility of HbS is a mixture of $\alpha_2^G\beta_2^A$ plus $\alpha_2^A\beta_2^S$. The component migrating like HbC, and comprising 10 to 15 percent of the total, is a mixture of HbA_2 ($\alpha_2\delta_2$) and the hybrid molecule $\alpha_2^G\beta_2^S$.

When the cellulose acetate electrophoretic pattern suggests Sickle Cell Anemia but the patient is not anemic or a few clinical manifestations of Sickle Cell Disease, or has splenomegaly persisting into adulthood, there are two procedures that may be employed to establish the diagnosis. One is to perform citrate agar gel electrophoresis at pH6.4 (Fig. 2B). There are several versions of this technique that can be employed [17,18,19]. We now use one in which the same mylar backed cellulose acetate plates used for the standard electrophoresis are impregnated with the agar [19]. With this technique HbA and HbS are separated but the D or G hemoglobins migrate with HbA. Thus, a HbG-trait, appearing like Sickle Cell Trait at pH 8.6 but having a negative solubility test will have a citrate agar gel pattern identical with the normal. The sickle cell HbD_β will have a citrate agar pattern similar to that of Sickle Cell Trait, the component migrating like HbA being, in fact, HbD. The second procedure employed is to study the family. One parent should have a negative solubility test or sickle cell prep, despite the electrophoretic pattern of Sickle Cell Trait or other relatives may have HbD trait.

SICKLE CELL β-THALASSEMIA

Thalassemia is a genetic disease such that an individual who has one dose of the thalassemia gene has mild hypochromia and microcytosis, target cells, and amiso- and poikilocytosis; it looks a lot like iron deficiency, except that such patients do not respond to iron therapy and the serum iron concentration is elevated (see reference #20 for a review). The thalassemia trait is characterized by mean hemoglobin concentrations 2.5 grams percent below normal, which means that many of them have normal hemoglobin levels. On the other hand, they may have hemoglobin concentrations as low as 9 grams percent. The most pathognomonic finding is elevation of the proportion of HbA_2 present, normally comprising 2 to 3 percent of the total hemoglobin, to twice normal levels. Homozygosity for the thalassemia genes is easy to diagnose. Hepatosplenomegaly, severe hypochromic-microcytic anemia, with hemoglobins below 6 grams percent, and requirement of transfusions every three to four weeks characterize classical thalassemia major or Cooley's anemia.

Now, what happens if a person inherits a sickle gene from one parent and a thalassemia gene from the other? There are two possible electrophoretic patterns (Table 1). The simplest one possesses between 10 and 25 percent of HbA with the remainder HbS (excluding HbA_2 and F from consideration). That is the converse of sickle trait which contains 60 percent of HbA and 35 percent of HbS. Therefore, when one sees reversal of the A:S ratio one can say that the patient has Sickle

Cell Thalassemia, provided, of course, one has ascertained that the patient has not had a transfusion. A Sickle Cell Anemia patient who has received a transfusion may have a similar pattern. Sickle Cell Thalassemia individuals have 4 to 6 percent of HbA_2.

The second variety of Sickle Cell Thalassemia has no HbA at all. Persons with this type have 70 to 90 percent of S hemoglobin, and HbF may comprise 20 to 30 percent of the total hemoglobin. This kind appears identical to Sickle Cell Anemia, except that proportion of HbA_2 is twice the normal level. This type of Sickle Cell Thalassemia should be suspected when persons having predominantly HbS also have splenomegaly in adulthood, inordinate hypochromia and microcytosis, or when family studies reveal that only one parent has Sickle Cell Trait. In this case the proportion of HbA_2 in that parent should be measured or other stigmata of thalassemia should be sought.

Those two forms of Sickle Cell β-thalassemia are reflections of two different β-thalassemia genes. The form possessing a minor amount of HbA is the type found most often in American and African Negroes. It is referred to as the African or β+ type. The thalassemia manifesting no HbA when in combination with $\underline{Hb_\beta}^S$ is referred to as the Mediterranean, the Ferrara, or the β^o type. It is the type found most often in persons of southern Mediterranean ancestry. In both types the synthesis of beta chains is suppressed completely or partially. In both the thalassemia genes is an allele or closely linked to the $\underline{Hb_\beta}$ structural locus.

SICKLE CELL HEREDITARY PERSISTENCE OF FETAL HEMOGLOBIN

Fetal hemoglobin comprises 75 percent of the hemoglobin at birth. It falls to less than 2 percent of the total hemoglobin in normal adults and in children beyond the first year of life. In some otherwise normal persons the HbF levels off at between 10 and 30 percent HbF, the remainder being HbA. They do not have thalassemia, they are not anemic, their red cell life span is normal, as is their red cell morphology; they simply have a persistance of fetal hemoglobin. This phenotype is determined by a single gene. Homozygotes for this gene have only fetal hemoglobin with no HbA and no HbA_2 [21].

A person who inherits one of these hereditary persistance of fetal hemoglobin genes from one parent and from the other a $\underline{Hb_{\beta}}^{S}$ gene has an electrophoretic pattern that is composed of 10 to 30 percent, generally 20 to 30 percent, of HbF and approximately 70 to 90 percent of HbS; it looks for all the world like Sickle Cell Anemia by electrophoresis. Yet, these individuals likewise have no anemia; their red cell life span is reputed to be normal, and their reticulocytes counts are normal. It is very important to differentiate this entity from a mild case of Sickle Cell Anemia, because of the very different prognosis and because of the different implications for genetic counseling. Sickle Cell HPFH can be diagnosed by studying the family to see if someone else in the family has a persistent high fetal hemoglobin trait. That is generally evident simply from the electrophoretic pattern.

A second option is the Kleihauer-Betke test [22]. This test provides a measure of the amount of fetal hemoglobin in individual cells. The test is executed by fixing a film of blood in 85 percent alcohol and then soaking the fixed film in a citrate acid-phosphate buffer at pH 3.2 to 3.4. The pH is very critical. Under these conditions adult hemoglobin, be it HbA or HbS is washed out of the cells and leaves behind the fetal hemoglobin which is then visible when the cells are stained with eosin. Cells that had contained only adult hemoglobin appear as ghosts, whereas those containing appreciable amounts of HbF are darkly stained.

Normally only 1 in a 100 or so of the erythrocytes contain HbF; the rest are ghosts. In Sickle Cell Anemia blood containing, say, 10 percent of fetal hemoglobin approximately 10 percent of the cells are stained, which is to say, in Sickle Cell Anemia the fetal hemoglobin is concentrated within a small clone of cells. In sickle cell - persistent fetal hemoglobin syndrome the HbF is distributed in most or all of the cells. Therefore, if the subject has 30 percent of HbF, every cell contains 30 percent of fetal hemoglobin. Presumably this amount of HbF in each cell is sufficient to prevent sickling under physiologic conditions, whereas in Sickle Cell Anemia a majority of the cells have no HbF, thus allowing these cells to sickle easily [23].

In summary, the diagnosis of Sickle Cell Anemia is generally easily made when the electrophoretic pattern is correlated with the clinical and hematologic findings. There remain a small group of patients, generally young children, who do not have the customary history of repeated crises and who have approximately 10 grams per 100 ml of hemoglobin. In these additional effort must be expended to exclude the three entities discussed above. In both the Howard University and Michigan Sickle Cell Centers we routinely measure the HbA_2 level and perform a citrate agar gel electrophoresis on each new patient in order to minimize the odds of misdiagnosis.

FUNCTIONAL MUTANTS OF HEMOGLOBIN

Genetic structural mutations may alter the function of hemoglobin in still other ways. On such class of mutants are the Hemoglobins M in which large amounts of methemoglobin are present [24]. This pigment, in which the iron is oxidized to the ferric state, is normally reduced to very low amounts by the methemoglobin reducing enzymes of the erythrocyte. The methemoglobin concentration may be increased in the blood either because oxidative chemicals have produced it in excess of the reductive capacity, or because of an inherited lack of the reductive enzymes. In the latter case the affected person's parents are asymptomatic heterozygotes and free of methemoglobin. But methemoglobin can also be due to structural alteration of either the alpha or the beta polypeptide chains. In these cases approximately 25 to 30 percent of the total pigment is so-call HbM. The sturctural lesion is in the proximity of the heme moiety of either the alpha or beta chains.

The heme group lies in a crevice of each polypeptide chain between two helical regions, the D and E helices. The iron atom of the heme group makes a coordinate bond with the imidazole groups of residues 58, in the D-helix, and 87 in the E helix of the alpha chain and, respectively, at positions 63 and 92 of the beta polypeptide chains. Structural mutants in which one of these histidines is substituted by tyrosine are summarized in Figure 5.

Hemoglobin M Substitutions

Alpha Chains

A	58	87
α	His . . Heme . . His	
M-Boston	58	87
α	Tyr —— Heme . . His	
M-Iwate	58	87
α	His . . Heme —— Tyr	

Beta Chains

A	63	92
β	His . . Heme . . His	
M-Saskatoon	63	92
β	Tyr —— Heme . . His	
M-Hyde Park	63	92
β	His . . Heme —— Tyr	

Fig. 5. Schematic diagram showing the location of the amino acid substitution in the various Hb M *mutants.*

The tyrosine so alters the reactivity of the iron atom that the iron remains oxidized and is not responsive to methemoglobin reductase. In these mutants a parent or offspring is often also affected. Approximately one third of observed cases are new mutations, so the value of the familial distribution is limited.

Another class of mutants are those in which the amino acid substitution makes the molecule unstable, either to conditions within the erythrocyte or to heating *in vitro* [25]. The molecular lesion is the result of conformational disturbances due either to the insertion of a charged amino acid in a hydrophobic region of the molecule, or to a large amino acid in a crowded region causing steric disturbances. Heterozygotes may have significant hemolytic anemia, especially after exposure to certain oxidative drugs. Incubation with oxidative dye may result in stainable inclusion bodies in the erythrocytes [26]. Heat denaturation is evaluated by heating a buffered solution at 50°C for one hour. The homolysate is centrifuged to spin down denatured hemoglobin and the absorbance of the supernate is measured. If the absorbance decreases more than 10 percent below the pre-heating value, an unstable hemoglobin is present, even though the electrophoretic pattern is normal. Another technique employs heating at 37°C in the presence of isopropanol [27].

Amino acid substitutions may alter the oxygen affinity of the molecule. In a number of mutants [28] the abnormal hemoglobin has increased affinity for oxygen, which is to say, the oxygen dissociation curve is displaced to the left, having a diminished P_{50}. These individuals have erythrocytosis, with hemoglobin concentrations as high as 23 gm percent. The electrophoretic pattern may be normal, so measurement of the oxyhemoglobin dissociation curve is necessary to exclude this possibility. These amino acids are generally the result of amino acid substitutions in the so-called $\alpha_1\beta_2$ subunit surface. This is the surface between the two $\alpha\beta$ dimers into which the hemoglobin molecule naturally dissociates. The unstable hemoglobins are frequently due to amino acid substitutions in the so-called $\alpha_1\beta_1$ surface, between the two chains within an $\alpha\beta$ dimer.

Lastly, thus far all of the abnormal hemoglobins that I have discussed have been the result of single amino acid substitutions in one polypeptide chain or another. An increasing number of variants have more complex abnormalities. For instance, Hb Leiden [27] has a deletion of the glutamic acid residue at β6 or 7 and Hb Gun Hill [30] is due to a deletion of five residues in the vicinity of β87-92. Hb Grady [31] on the other hand is an insertion of three residues between positions 118 and 119. A number of Hb Lepores have been described [5] in which a portion of the non-alpha polypeptide chain at the free amino end has the sequence of delta chains, whereas the remaining portion toward the carboxyl end have beta chain sequences. Hb Wayne [32] is a frame shift mutant in which the last three amino acids of the alpha chain are replaced by eight additional residues. All of these mutants are explainable as products of unequal crossing over. Hb Constant Spring [33] has the entire sequence of the alpha chain plus thirty-one (31) additional residues. It can be deduced from Hb Wayne that this mutant is the result of a base-pair substitution in the chain terminating codon of the alpha chain.

Human hemoglobins continues to be a sensitive selective system for detecting genetic variability in man.

ACKNOWLEDGEMENT

The author is grateful for the technical assistance of Floretta J. Reynolds.

REFERENCES

1. Neel, J.V. *The Inheritance Of The Sickling Phenomenon, With Particular Reference To Sickle Cell Disease.* Blood 6:389-412, 1951.

2. Pauling, L., Itano, H.A., Singer, S.J., and Wells, I.C. *Sickle Cell Anemia, A Molecular Disease.* Science 110:543-548, 1949.

3. Itano, H.A. and Neel, J.V. *A New Inherited Abnormality Of Human Hb.* Proc. Nat. Acad. Sci. 36: 613, 1950.

4. Winter, W.P. and Rucknagel, D.L. *Peptide Mapping Of Hemoglobin.* In: Schmidt, A.M., Huisman, T.H.J.,

and Lehmann, H., Eds. *The Detection Of Hemoglobinopathies.* Cleveland, Oh., C.R.C. Press. pp. 51-70, 1974.

5. Huisman, T.H.J. *Normal And Abnormal Human Hemoglobins.* Adv. Clin. Chem. 15:149-253, 1972.

6. Lehmann, H., and Carrell, R.W. *Differences Between* α- and β-chain *Mutants Of Human Haemoglobin And Between* α- and β-*thalassemia. Possible Duplication Of the* α-chain *Gene.* Brit. Med. J. 4: 748-750, 1968.

7. Hollan, S.R., Szelenzi, J.G., Brimhall, B., Duerst, M., Jones, R.T., Koler, R.D., and Stocklen, Z. *Multiple Alpha Chain Loci For Human Haemoglobins* HbJ-Bada *and* HbG-Pest. Nature 235:47-50, 1972.

8. Dublin, P.A., Jr., Cates, M., and Rucknagel, D.L. *Bimodality Of The Proportion Of* HbGα-Philadelphia *Suggesting Heterogeneity In The Number Of Hemoglobin Alpha Chain Loci.* Ped. Res. 8:388, 1974.

9. Rucknagel, D.L. and Winter, W.P. *Duplication Of Structural Genes For Hemoglobin Alpha And Beta Chains In Man.* Ann. Y.Y. Acad. Sci. In press.

10. Schroeder, W.A., et. al. *Evidence For Multiple Structural Genes For The* γ *Chain Of Human Fetal Hemoglobin.* Proc. Nat. Acad. Sci. U.S. 60:537-544, 1968.

11. Huisman, T.H.J., Schroeder, W.A., Bannister, W.H., and Grech, J.L. *Evidence For Four Nonallelic Structural Genes For The* γ *Chain Of Human Fetal Hemoglobin.* Biochem. Genet. 7:131-139, 1972.

12. Boyer, S.H., Rucknagel, D.L., Weatherall, D.J., and Watson-Williams, E.J. *Further Evidence For Linkage Between The* β and δ *Loci Governing Human Hemoglobin And The Population Dynamics Of Linked*

Genes. Amer. J. Hum. Genet. 15:438-448, 1963.

13. Pearson, H.A., and Moore, M.M. *Human Hemoglobin Gene Linkage: Report Of A Family With Hemoglobin* β_2*, Hemoglobin* S., *And* β *Thalassemia, Including A Probable Crossover Between Thalassemia And Delta Loci.* Amer. J. Hum. Genet. 17:125-132, 1965.

14. Schmidt, R.M. and Wilson, S.M. *Standardization In Detection Of Abnormal Hemoglobins. Solubility Tests For Hemoglobin* S. J.A.M.A. 225:1225-1230, 1973.

15. McKusick, V.A. *Mendelian Inheritance In Man, Third Edition.* Baltimore, Johns Hopkins Press, 1971.

16. Rucknagel, D.L. *The Genetics Of Sickle Cell Anemia And Related Syndromes.* Arch. Int. Med. 133:595-606, 1974.

17. Robinson, A.R., Robson, M., Harrison, A.P., and Zuelzer, W.W. *A New Technique For Differentiation Of Hemoglobin.* J. Lab. Clin. Med. 50:745-752, 1957.

18. Marder, V.J. and Conley, C.L. *Electrophoresis Of Hemoglobin On Agar Gels.* Bulletin Of The Johns Hopkins Hospital 105:2, pp. 77-88, 1959.

19. Schneider, R.G. *Identification Of Hemoglobins By Electrophoresis.* In: Schmidt, R.M., Huisman, T.H.J., and Lehmann, H., eds. Cleveland, Oh., C.R.C. Press, pp. 11-14, 1974.

20. Weatherall, D.J., and Clegg, J.B. *The Thalassemia Syndromes, Second Ed.*, Oxford, Blackwell Publ. pp. 374, 1972.

21. Wheeler, J.T., Krevans, J.R. *The Homozygous State Of Persistent Fetal Hemoglobin And The Interaction Of Persistent Fetal Hemoglobin With*

Thalassemia. Bull. Johns Hopkins Hosp. 109: 217-233, November, 1961.

22. Huisman, T.H.J. *Human Hemoglobins, In Yanis, J.J.*, ed. *Biochemical Methods In Red Cell Genetics*. New York, Academic Press, pp. 391-530, 1969.

23. Shepard, M.K., Weatherall, D.J., and Conley, C.L. *Semi-quantitative Estimation Of The Distribution Of Fetal Hemoglobin In Red Cell Populations* Johns Hopkins Hospital Bulletin: 110-111, 293-310, 1962.

24. Jaffe, E.R., and Heller, P. *Methemoglobinemia In Man*. Progr. Hemat. 4:48-71, 1964.

25. Carrell, R.W., and Lehmann, H. *The Unstable Haemoglobin Haemolytic Anemias*. Sem. Hematol. 6: 116-132, 1969.

26. Papayannopoulos, T., and Stamatoyannopoulos, G. *Stains For Inclusion Bodies*. In: Schmidt, R.M. Huisman, T.H.J., and Lehmann, H., eds. *The Detection Of Hemoglobinopathies*, Cleveland, Oh., C.R.C. Press, pp. 32-38, 1974.

27. Carrell, R.W., and Kay, R. *A Simple Method For The Detection Of Unstable Haemoglobins*. Brit. J. Haemat. 23:615-619, 1972.

28. Stamatoyannopoulos, G., Bellingham, A.J., Lenfant, C., and Finch, C.A. *Abnormal Hemoglobins With High And Low Oxygen Affinity*. Ann. Rev. Med. 22:221-234, 1971.

29. DeJong, W.W.W., Went, L.N., and Bernini, L.F. *Haemoglobin Leiden: Deletion Of* β6 *or* 7 *Glutamic Acid*. Nature 220: 788-790, 1968.

30. Bradley, T.B., Jr., Wohl, R.C., and Rieder, R.F. *Hemoglobin Gun Hill: Deletion Of Five Amino*

And Residues And Impaired Heme-globin Binding. Sci. 157:1581-1583, 1967.

31. Huisman, T.H.J., Wilson, J.B., Gravely, M., and Hubbard, M. *Hemoglobin Grady: The First Example Of A Variant With Elongated Chains Due To Insertion Of Residues.* Proc. Nat. Acad. Sci., U.S., 71:3270-3273, 1974.

32. Seid-Akhavan, M., Winter, W.P., Abramson, R.K., and Rucknagel, D.L. *Hemoglobin Wayne: A Frameshift Variant Occurring In Two Distinct Forms.* Blood 40:927 (Abstr.), 1972.

33. Clegg, J.B., Weatherall, D.J., and Milner, P.F. *Haemoglobin Constant Spring: A Chain Termination Mutant?* Nature 234:337-340, 1971.

VARIATIONS IN THE SYNTHESIS AND CELLULAR CONTENT OF STRUCTURALLY DISTINCT HUMAN HEMOGLOBINS

Ronald F. Rieder, M.D.

INTRODUCTION

Human hemoglobins present a wide spectrum of normal and abnormal variations in the structure of the globin or protein portion of the molecule [1]. Some of these diverse hemoglobin types such as HbF ($\alpha_2\gamma_2$), and HbA$_2$ ($\alpha_2\delta_2$) are normal forms which are produced at stages of human development and/or in amounts which differ from that of the major adult component, HbA ($\alpha_2\beta_2$). These normal variants have "non-α" chains determined by genes which are distinctive from the gene specifying the β chain of HbA. Other types of variants such as HbS (β^6 gly-val, i.e., valine is substituted for glycine in position 6 of the β chain), HbG Philadelphia (α68 asn-lys) and Hb Lepore ($\alpha_2\delta\beta_2$), constitute a sizeable group of mutant proteins having amino acid substitutions, deletions, or fusion chains. The many abnormal hemoglobins are found in greatly differing proportions in the blood of affected subjects.

The problem of the differential regulation of human hemoglobin synthesis has received much attention in recent years. In part this interest has been generated because a group of important disease states, the hemoglobinopathies, is associated with structurally abnormal hemoglobins [2]. In addition, a widespread group of syndromes, termed the thalassemias, results from defects in the synthetic rate of structurally normal globin chains [3]. A better understanding of the factors controlling hemoglobin synthesis and of the relationship of structure to synthetic rate should prove to be of great clinical significance, possibly even clarifying the pathogenesis of some of the disorders and/or suggesting useful therapeutic measures. Moreover, the wide variety of structural alterations found in these proteins, the diversity in amounts of each type produced, the ease of obtaining purified components, and the single-mindedness of the red cell in synthesizing almost exclusively hemoglobin, render the human erythrocyte precursor an especially interesting system for studying the effects of structural mutations on protein biosynthesis. This review will briefly summarize some of the observations that have been made, and the information currently available, regarding the control of the differential synthesis of normal and abnormal human hemoglobins.

MECHANISM OF HEMOGLOBIN SYNTHESIS

Protein synthesis is a multi-step process and regulation of the rates of production of the different types of normal and abnormal globin chains could theoretically occur at any of several stages. In the cell nucleus the messenger RNA for a given protein is synthesized upon the corresponding gene during the process of transcription. The specific nucleotide sequence of the DNA of the gene acts as a template which directs the sequential linking of mononucleotides into the polynucleotide mRNA through the action of the enzyme RNA polymerase. Modifying factors which affect the availability of the template, the attachment of the enzyme, or its activity upon the template, may alter the rate of mRNA productio There is evidence that after synthesis certain mRNA's may undergo cleavage from a larger precursor molecule (HnRNA) [5]. A length of polyadenylate (poly A) whose function is not well understood, is added to the 3' end of the mRNA which must then be transferred into the cyt plasm [6]. No information is presently available relatin specific nuclear processes to differential synthesis of globin chains.

In the cytoplasm the messenger RNA may be processe further by removal of a portion of the poly A sequence The mRNA then acts in the cytoplasm as a specific template for polypeptide chain assembly in the process of translation. The linking of the various amino acids by peptide bonding takes place on mRNA multi-ribosomal complexes (polyribosomes). The process of polypeptide assembly requires the presence of a series of proteins acting as initiation and chain elongation factors, t-RNA's, which bring the various amino acids to the polyribosomes for correct sequential linkage, GTP, ATP, and amino acid-tRNA synthetases, which attach the amino acids to specific t-RNA's [8]. After the completion of the linking of the amino acids, the newly synthesized peptide chains are released from the polyribosomes, heme is added, and the hemoglobin tetramer is formed. Specificity of certain initiation factors, elongation factors, or tRNA's for different globin chains or perturbations in any of these or other multiple cytoplasmic factors could affect polypeptide chain production, conceivably in a manner specific enough to cause a differential rate of translation of the various types of globins. Differential stability of mRNA could also influence globin chain synthesis in a specific manner. However, no well-defined selective mechanism affecting the synthesis of the various types of non-α chains has been demonstrated as yet. Some specificity in regard to α versus β synthesis is suggested by the finding that α chain production tends to decline more rapidly than β chain synthesis during prolonged incubation of human reticulocytes in vitro [9]. It also appears that the initiation of translation of α globin mRNA (Attachment to ribosomes) may be less efficient than for β mRNA [10]. In addition, it has been shown that manipulation of the mRNA concentration can alter the α/β globin synthesis ratio in cell-free experiments [11]. Thus there does appear to be a degree of non-equivalence in the cytoplasmic processes resulting in α and β globin synthesis.

HEMOGLOBIN A_2 AND RELATED HEMOGLOBINS

The δ chain of hemoglobin A_2 differs from the β chain of hemoglobin A in only 10 out of the 146 amino acids which constitute each of the polypeptides. Despite the structural similarity of the two globins and the fact that the genes determining their production are closely linked, or perhaps even contiguous on the same chromosome, there is a marked inequality in the synthesis of the two polypeptides, HbA_2 occurring in amounts 2-3 percent of HbA. The cause of this great disparity in synthesis is not understood. In addition to the smaller total δ chain production per erythrocyte, there is a more rapid rate of decline in δ chain synthesis than β chain synthesis as the erythroid cell matures. Thus at the reticulocyte stage δ chains are no longer produced while some β chain synthesis continues [12,13].

The Lepore-type hemoglobins are a group of abnormal hemoglobins which have a $\delta\beta$ "fusion" chain as the non-α chain. These "fusion" polypeptides have a sequence of amino acids of variable length extending from the N-terminal end which is "δ-like" while the remaining portion of the chain extending to the C-terminal end is "β-chain-like." The different fusion chains that have been described are probably the result of variably misplaced synapses with unequal crossing-over occurring during meiosis [14]. Several Lepore-type hemoglobins with different cross-over points have been found [15]. The hemoglobins Lepore occur in heterozygotes in amounts intermediate (about 15% of total hemoglobin) between that normally found for HbA and HbA_2.

The formation of a Lepore gene implies the possibility of a simultaneous formation of the corresponding "anti-Lepore" or $\beta\delta$ fusion gene on the opposite chromatid. Hb Miyada and Hb P Congo are abnormal variants which contain the anticipated $\beta\delta$ fusion chain ("β-like" at N-terminus, "δ-like" at C-terminus). These hemoglobins also occur in amounts equal to 15-20% of the red cell hemoglobin [16,17]. Similar to HbA_2, the Lepore hemoglobins and Hb Miyada are no longer synthesized at the reticulocyte stage of red cell development [13,18,19,20].

The basis for these anomalies of synthesis of δ, $\delta\beta$, and $\beta\delta$ chains is not apparent. The translation rates (time required to assemble a single chain on the ribosome) of β, δ, and $\delta\beta$ chains have been examined and appear similar [13,21]. It is possible that the stabilit of the mRNA's for these globins is decreased compared to β globin mRNA. This instability would explain the more rapid cessation of synthesis of δ and "δ-like" chains in the more mature erythroid elements where no mRNA production occurs, as well as the observed rapid loss of synthetic capacity of marrow cells for these globins upon prolonged incubation in vitro [21]. A stabilizing function for the poly A sequence of rabbit globin mRNA has been proposed recently [22]. However, the structural basis for a differential stability of the human globin mRNA's is not apparent. It would not seem likely to lie exclusively in a loss due to crossing over of either the poly A region or another untranslated sequence found only at either the 5' or 3' end of the β globin mRNA since both δβ and βδ chains display the same synthetic peculiarities. Clegg and Weatherall, however, have suggested that stabilizing regions may occur at both ends of the β mRNA[23]. Similarly, the relative repression of δ chain synthesis compared to β chain production at all stages of erythrocyte maturation remains unexplained but might also be due to instability of δ globin mRNA due to absence of the untranslated stabilizing regions found in β globin mRNA. Isolation, quantitation and characterization of δ or δβ globin mRNA might provide additional insight into these problems.

FETAL HEMOGLOBINS

The γ chain of HbF differs from the β chain of HbA by 39 amino acids [24]. HbF appears early in human fetal development and at birth comprises 60-70% of the circulating hemoglobin of the infant. Synthesis of the γ globin chain declines swiftly after birth and by 6-9 months of age the level of HbF is reduced to about 1% of the circulating hemoglobin. This small amount of HbF constitutes the normal level found in older children and adults.

Studies by Schroeder and associates have demonstrated that humans possess two closely linked genes for γ chains [25]. Two forms of γ globin chains are produced, Gγ and Aγ, and differ only in having either glycine or alanine at position 136. The ratio of the Gγ:Aγ chains present in HbF changes from 7:3 at birth to 2:3 by 5 months of age.

High levels of HbF persist past infancy in the blood of individuals with some forms of thalassemia [3], in a high proportion of patients with sickle cell anemia, and in certain syndromes associated with chromosomal abnormalities [26]. Reappearance of high levels of HbF in later life can occur in subjects with various acquired disorders including chronic myelogenous leukemia of childhood [27], aplastic anemia [28], and paroxysmal nocturnal hemoglobinuria. In all these disease states, HbF is heterogeneously distributed among the erythrocytes. Some cells contain almost no HbF while others contain a great deal. It is likely that the persistance or reactivation on HbF synthesis in these conditions is associated with a continued or renewed proliferation of clones of erythropoietic cells which are distinct from the clones producing mainly the adult variety of hemoglobin. Marked variations in the Gγ:Aγ ratios have been noted in the various disease states mentioned above [29,30].

In a group of disorders termed hereditary persistance of fetal hemoglobin (HPFH), elevated levels of HbF continue into adult life, hematological abnormalities are slight or absent, and HbF is evenly distributed among the red blood cells [31]. In the form of the disorder seen in Negroes the β and δ chain genes appear to be deleted from the affected chromosome so that heterozygotes have low levels of HbA and A_2 and homozygotes produce only HbF [32]. In the Greek form of HPFH, heterozygotes possess lower levels of HbF than in the Negro type [33]. In addition, in the Greek syndrome the affected chromosome appears to direct some β and δ synthesis although at a lower level than in normal subjects. Analysis of the HbF in the Greek disorder indicates that only Aγ chains are produced [34]. The Negro form of the syndrome seems to be more genetically varied so that subjects have been described with only Gγ, or both Gγ and Aγ chains in HbF [34].

An additional variety of HPFH has recently been described in association with Hb Kenya ($\alpha_2\gamma\beta_2$) [35,36].

This abnormal hemoglobin has a $\gamma\beta$ fusion polypeptide as the non-α chain. Hb Kenya is thus analogous to Hb Lepore and probably results from a cross-over occurring between the $A\gamma$ gene and the β gene somewhere between the nucleotides determining residues 81 and 86 [35,36]. Hb Kenya comprises about 16% of the total hemoglobin in hemolysates and HbF levels are elevated to 5-10% and contain only $G\gamma$ chains. HbA_2 levels are reduced. As a result of the discovery and analysis of Hb Kenya, the normal chromosomal gene sequence appears to be: $G\gamma$-$A\gamma$-δ-β. The Kenya chromosome has probably undergone a deletion of the entire δ gene and portions of the $A\gamma$ and β genes to give the sequence $G\gamma$-$\gamma\beta$.

The combination of gene deletion and increased fetal hemoglobin production seen in these syndromes of HPFH suggests the possibility that operator genes [37], which are contiguous to the structural gene and which may normally suppress γ chain synthesis after fetal life, are lost along with the deleted structural genes. Elaborate hypotheses have been constructed to explain the observations but further evidence is needed [38].

The ε globin chains of hemoglobin Gower I, (ε_4) and Gower II, ($\alpha_2\varepsilon_2$), are normally produced only during the first trimester of intrauterine life [39]. The factors responsible for the switching on and off of embryonic globin synthesis are not known.

ABNORMAL HEMOGLOBINS

The wide variation in the amounts of the different abnormal hemoglobins found in the peripheral blood of heterozygotes is shown in Table I. The range of values extends from 58% for Hb Hijiyama [40] to less than 3% for Hb Constant Spring [59] and Hb Bushwick [60]. In general, structurally abnormal hemoglobins occur in smaller amounts than HbA.

Hemoglobin S has been the most intensively studied of the mutant hemoglobins. Although HbS always occurs in smaller amounts than HbA in the blood of AS heterozygotes (sickle cell trait), a significant variation in the quantity of the abnormal hemoglobin found in sickle cell trait has been frequently observed [46,47,61].

TABLE 1. *PROPORTION OF ABNORMAL HEMOGLOBIN IN HETEROZYGOTES*

Name	*Substitution*	*%*	*Reference No.*
Hijiyama	β120 lys-glu	58	40
J Baltimore	β 16 gly-asp	44	41
G Honolulu	α 30 Glu-glu	50	42
J Tongariki	α115 ala-asp	40-47	43
G Phila-delphia	α 68 asn-lys	33-45	44,45
S	β 6 glu-val	27-45	46,47,48
E	β 26 glu-lys	25-30	44,50
Zurich	β 63 his-arg	19-27	51,52,53
Koln	β 98 val-met	11-14	54
Hasharon	α 47 asp-his	14-19	55,56,57
J Toronto	α 5 ala-asp	20	58
Constant Spring	α	2.5	59
Bushwick	β 74 gly-val	<2	60

There is some evidence that within families the cellular content of HbS tends to cluster suggesting the possibility of genetically controlled auxiliary factors affecting the amount of synthesis of the mutant hemoglobin [47,48]. However, "clustering" of HbS levels in individual families has not been uniformly noted [62]. Recently, decreased stability with increased turnover rate of HbS has been suggested as being partially responsible for the unusually low levels of the mutant protein found in some heterozygous individuals [63]. Further study of this phenomenon is indicated as prior investigations did not indicate increased destruction of HbS [64,65,66].

Non-genetic factors such as iron deficiency and megaloblastic anemia can lower the level of an abnormal hemoglobin relative to HbA [67,68].

The presence of another hemoglobin apparently can influence the cellular content of a given mutant hemoglobin. Subjects heterozygous for HbA and HbJ-Baltimore (β^{16} gly-asp) generally have about 40% HbJ. In the presence of the β^{S} gene, absolute synthesis of βJ Baltimore appears to be increased. Weatherall has reported that

S-J heterozygotes can possess up to 70% HbJ with hematocrit values and red blood cell indices similar to A-J heterozygotes [41].

An excellent example of markedly decreased synthesis of a globin chain due to a structural abnormality is seen in HbE. Subjects with HbE trait generally have 25-30% abnormal hemoglobin [49,50]. Although there is evidence of slightly increased turnover of HbE the small amount of HbE (25-30%) found in AE heterozygotes appears to be mainly a result of defective synthesis of β^{E} [50].

In contrast to the decreased production of β^{E}, increased synthesis of a mutant β chain relative to β^{A} occurs in subjects with Hb Gun Hill ($\alpha_2\beta_2$ 92-97 deleted)[69]. This distorted hemoglobin lacks heme on the β chains and is unstable. The increased degradation of the mutant portein results in cellular levels of Hb Gun Hill which are considerably below the percentage of HbA (about 30% of total) [70]. However, studies of globin chain synthesis in vitro and in vivo indicated that β^{GH} is actually produced in greater amounts than β^{A} [70,71].

Under normal physiological circumstances the synthesis of α and β chains is approximately equal so that no excess of either polypeptide is produced. Unbalanced synthesis is characteristic of the several thalassemia syndromes which are discussed below [3]. In other disorders including the structural hemoglobinopathies, equal amounts of α and β (or β + γ) globins are produced. Recently, however, studies of the synthesis of Hb Leiden ($\alpha_2\beta^{6 \text{ or } 7 \text{ glu deleted}}$) in marrow and peripheral blood, in vitro, have demonstrated a marked relative deficiency of β chain production [72,73]. The β^{A}/α and β^{Leiden}/α synthetic ratios were 0.35 and 0.25 respectively with a total β/α ratio of 0.6. Such marked imbalance in chain synthesis is distinctly unusual in the absence of a thalassemia gene.

The several examples detailed above of defective or altered synthesis of the structurally abnormal globins remain unexplained. Investigations of the functioning of subcellular mechanisms of globin synthesis in the presence of abnormal globins have been limited to the cytoplasm. Studies of globin chain translation rates have been performed on several abnormal hemoglobins

S [74], C [74], Gun Hill [71], Riverdale-Bronx [75], Leiden [76] and K Woolwich [77]. No evidence for disturbances in the ribosomal assembly of these abnormal polypeptides has been obtained.

UNSTABLE HEMOGLOBINS

There is a constantly enlarging list of human hemoglobin mutants which are classified as unstable [78]. These variants have amino acid changes involving critical areas of the hemoglobin molecule which, under minimal stress, result in marked alteration or dissolution of the normal precisely ordered three-dimensional structure of globin [79].

Studies of incorporation of radioactive tracers in vivo and in vitro, by peripheral blood reticulocytes and bone marrow cells obtained from heterozygotes, have indicated that several of the unstable hemoglobins have a faster turnover rate than HbA. This phenomenon was first suggested in studies of Hb Zurich [52]. Subsequently similar observations have been made on hemoglobins Gun Hill [70,71], Riverdale-Bronx [80,66], Koln [54,81], Hammersmith [82], Bristol [83], Genova [84], Leiden [72,73], Bushwick [60], and Abraham Lincoln [85]. The more rapid destruction of the unstable hemoglobins explains the reduced amounts of those mutants often found in blood. The most striking example of differential turnover of hemoglobins has been noted in association with Hb Bushwick. This unstable variant is synthesized in vitro by reticulocytes at a rate no less than 30-40% of HbA but is found in only trace amounts in mature erythrocytes [60]. Accompanying the dissolution of the abnormal hemoglobin with loss of the unstable abnormal globin chains, the normal complementary chains in the tetramer are released and often appear free within the erythrocyte [71]. These released chains may have an influence on globin chain synthesis. Feedback inhibition of normal β chain synthesis by β chains released by degradation of the unstable α chain mutant Hb Ann Arbor (α_2 80 leu-argβ_2) has been suggested [86]. However, no such inhibition of synthesis of the complementary globin chain has been observed with Hb Bushwick or several other unstable hemoglobins.

HEMOGLOBINS WITH ABNORMAL α CHAINS

Although fewer in number than the known β chain mutations a sizeable group of α chain mutations have been recognized [1]. Lehmann and Carrell first pointed out that while most β chain mutants (unstable hemoglobins excepted) make up 35-45% of the total erythrocyte hemoglobin in heterozygotes, most hemoglobins with mutations in the α chain occur in the range of only 20-25% [87]. Those authors suggested that if there were two non-allelic α globin loci, only one of 4 α globin genes might be altered in an individual heterozygous for an α chain mutant, and thus the proportion of the abnormal hemoglobin would be low, i.e., approximately 25%.

Evidence supporting the concept of two α chain loci has been obtained in some racial groups of man. A Hungarian family has been reported in which 2 abnormal α chain variants, HbJ-Buda and HbG-Pest, were segregating [88]. One individual possessed both abnormal hemoglobins in addition to HbA. Duplicated α chain genes also appear to exist in some subjects from Southeast Asia. Homozygotes for Hb Constant Spring, an α chain mutant, also exhibit HbA [89]. However, such duplication of the α chain loci is apparently not universal in humans. Subjects homozygous for the α chain mutant HbJ Tongariki possess 100% abnormal hemoglobin [43]. Other evidence suggesting that not all humans carry duplicated α chain loci comes from a consideration of certain α chain mutants occurring in high quantities (Table 1). In some families, subjects with HbG Philadelphia exhibit this abnormal hemoglobin in amounts about 45% while in other families, individuals have only 30-33% of that α chain variant [44,45]. Rucknagel [90] has pointed out that if the gene for the α G-Philadelphia chain were situated on a chromosome bearing only a single α locus, a heterozygote would have either about 33% or slightly below 50% abnormal hemoglobin depending on whether the "trans" chromosome bore one or two normal α^A loci. There appears to be some direct genetic evidence supporting the concept that the α G-Philadelphia gene is situated on a chromosome with a single α locus [90]. A woman heterozygous for α thalassemia and HbG Philadelphia has been found to synthesize only HbH and HbG Philadelphia [90,76].

THALASSEMIA

The thalassemia syndromes are a group of disorders characterized by deficient hemoglobinization of erythro cytes due to absent or reduced synthesis of either the α or β globin chains (α thalassemia and β thalassemia)[3] Production of the opposite globin chain persists at a nearly normal rate with resultant imbalance in α/β synthesis and accumulation of the unaffected chain [91,92,93,94]. The excess chains cannot form a stable tetramer denature readily, and precipitate to form intracellular inclusion bodies [95]. These inclusion bodies may damage the erythrocyte membrane resulting in increased hemolysis [96]. Increased amounts of HbF are commonly seen in the blood of patients with β-thalassemia but the structure of the globin produced in thalassemia is normal ex cept in subjects with the recently described form of α-thalassemia associated with Hb Constant Spring [59]. In that syndrome the reduced production of α Constant Spri leads to an imbalance in α/β synthesis with β globin ex cess.

The search for the molecular defect in the thalassemia disorders has attracted the participation of many laboratories which have contributed to steady progress in the understanding of these diseases. In vitro studies utilizing reticulocytes for incorporation of radioactive tracers into protein demonstrated unequal production of α and β globin chains confirming the clin cally suspected defects in hemoglobin synthesis in α- and β-thalassemia [91,92,93,94]. Investigations of the mechanism and kinetics of the initiation of globin chai assembly and of the process of mRNA translation reveale no differences between thalassemic and normal erythrocytes. The results suggested that in thalassemia the available globin mRNA functions qualitatively normally during the process of globin synthesis [97, 74, 98, 99]. Recent experiments utilizing cell-free systems to explore hemoglobin synthesis have indicated a deficient total activity of the mRNA for β-globin in β-thalassemia and a corresponding decreased activity of α chain mRNA in α-thalassemia [99,100,11,101]. Nucleic acid hybridization assays have confirmed that the actual quantity of the affected mRNA is decreased in these syndromes [102,103]. Thus these series of studies have tended to eliminate cytoplasmic processes as the basic source of the disordered globin chain synthesis in several of the thalassemic syndromes. It seems clear that attention will now turn to the examination of nuclear processes in the attempt to unravel the molecular pathology of thalassemia. Some progress seems to have been made already: DNA-DNA hybridization studies indicate absence or decrease of α chain genetic material in the severe form of homozygous α thalassemia characterized by absent α chain production, hydrops fetalis, and still birth [104,105]. Such precise information regarding the function of the involved genes is not yet available for β-thalassemia or the forms of α-thalassemia in which some α globin is produced. However, it seems likely that some sort of deficiency in the production or the processing of globin mRNA will be discovered to be the basic fault in those disorders.

SUMMARY

The many normal and abnormal structural variants of human hemoglobin occur in widely different amounts in peripheral erythrocytes. Accelerated destruction accounts for the decreased amounts of certain unstable mutant hemoglobins. Differences in synthetic rates appear to be responsible for most of the inequalities in the proportions of the other structural variants. The mechanisms for these quantitative differences are poorly understood. Elucidation of these processes will depend upon further advances in the knowledge of the regulation of mammalian protein synthesis in general. Hopefully, the continued application of the techniques of molecular biology to the examination of the human hemoglobinopathies will eventually lead to important therapeutic advances.

REFERENCES

1. Hunt, L.T. and Dayoff, M.O. *Table of Abnormal Human Globins in Atlas of Protein Sequence and Structure*, Volume 5, Supplement II, National Biomedical Research Foundation, Washington,1974.

2. Comings, D.E. *Erythrocyte Disorders - Anemias Related to Abnormal Globin in Hematology*, Williams, W.J., Beutler, E., Erslev, A.J., and Rundles, R. W. Editors. McGraw-Hill, New York, 1972, Chapters 46-49.

3. Weatherall, D.J. and Clegg, J.B. *The Thalassemia Syndromes*. Blackwell, Oxford, 1972.

4. Stein, G.S., Spelsberg, T.C. and Kleinsmith, L.J. *Nonhistone Chromosomal Proteins and Gene Regulation*. Science 183:817, 1974.

5. Williamson, R., Drewienkiewicz, C.E. and Paul, J. *Globin Messenger Sequences in High Molecular Weight RNA from Embryonic Mouse Liver*. Nature New Biology 241:66, 1973.

6. Braverman, G., Mendecki, J. and Lee, S.Y. *A Procedure for the Isolation of Mammalian Messenger Ribonucleic Acid*. Biochemistry 11:637, 1972.

7. Darnell, J.E., Jelinek, W.R. and Molloy, G.R. *Biogenesis of mRNA; Genetic Regulation in Mammalian Cells*. Science 181:1215, 1973.

8. Lipmann, F. *Polypeptide Chain Elongation in Protein Biosynthesis*. Science 164:1024, 1969.

9. Rieder, R.F. *Variation in β/α Synthesis Ratios in Thalassemia and Hemoglobinopathies*. Ann N.Y. Acad. Sci. 232:44, 1974.

10. Lodish, H.F. *Alpha and Beta Globin Messenger Ribonucleic Acid. Different Amounts and Rates of*

Initiation of Translation. J. Biol. Chem. 246: 7131, 1971.

11. Benz, E.J., Jr., Swerdlow, P.S. and Forget, B.G. *Globin Messenger RNA in Hemoglobin H Disease.* Blood 42:825, 1973.

12. Rieder, R.F. and Weatherall, D.J. *Studies on Hemoglobin Biosynthesis: Asynchronous Synthesis of Hemoglobin A and Hemoglobin A_2 by Erythrocyte Precursors.* J. Clin. Invest. 44:42, 1965.

13. Roberts, A.V., Weatherall, D.J. and Clegg, J.B. *The Synthesis of Human Haemoglobin A_2 During Erythroid Maturation.* Biochem. Biophys. Res. Comm. 47:81, 1972.

14. Baglioni, C. *The Fusion of Two Peptide Chains in Hemoglobin Lepore and its Interpretation as a Genetic Deletion.* Proc. Nat. Acad. Sci. 48: 1880, 1962.

15. Ostertag, W. and Smith, E.W. *Hemoglobin-Lepore Baltimore, A Third Type of a δβ Crossover, (δ^{50}, β^{86}).* Europ. J. Biochem. 10:371, 1969.

16. Ohta, Y., Yamaoka, K., Sumida, I., and Yanase, T. *Haemoglobin Miyada, α β-δ Fusion Peptide (Anti-Lepore) Type Discovered in a Japanese Family.* Nature New Biology 234:218, 1971.

17. Badr, F.M., Lorkin, P.A. and Lehmann, H. *Haemoglobin P-Nilotic Containing a β-δ Chain.* Nature New Biol. 242:107, 1973.

18. White, J.M., Lang, A., Lorkin, P.A. and Lehmann, H. *Synthesis of Haemoglobin Lepore.* Nature New Biology 235:208, 1972.

19. Gill, F., Atwater, J. and Schwartz, E. *Hemoglobin Lepore Trait: Globin Synthesis in Bone Marrow and Peripheral Blood.* Science 178:623, 1972.

20. Roberts, A.V., Clegg, J.B., Weatherall, D.J. and Ohta, Y. *Synthesis in vitro of Anti-Lepore Haemoglobin.* Nature New Biology 245:23, 1973.

21. Lang, A., White, J.M. and Lehmann, H. *Synthesis of Hb Lepore ($\alpha_2\delta\beta_2$). Influence of δ and β Nucleotide Sequence on Synthesis of δβ Chain.* Nature New Biology 240:268, 1972.

22. Huez, G., Marbaix, G., Hubert, E., Leclercq, M., Nudel, U., Soreq, H., Salomon, R., Lebleu, B., Revel, M., and Littauer, U.Z. *Role of the Polyadenylate Segment in the Translation of Globin Messenger RNA in Xenopus Oocytes.* Proc. Nat. Acad. Sci. (U.S.A.) 71:3143, 1974.

23. Clegg, J.B. and Weatherall, D.J. *β^o Thalassemia-time for a Reappraisal?* The Lancet 2:133, 1974.

24. Schroeder, W.A., Shelton, J.R., Shelton, J.B., Cormick, J. and Jones, R.T. *The Amino Acid Sequence of the γ Chain of Human Fetal Hemoglobin.* Biochemistry. 2:992, 1963.

25. Schroeder, W.A., Huisman, T.H.J., Shelton, J.R., Shelton, J.B., Kleihauer, E.F., Dozy, A.M. and Robberson, B. *Evidence for Multiple Structural Genes for the γ Chain of Human Fetal Hemoglobin.* Proc. Nat. Acad. Sci. U.S.A. 60:537, 1968.

26. Wilson, M.G., Schroeder, W.A., Graves, D.A. and Kach, V.D. *Hemoglobin Variations in D-trisomy Syndrome.* N.E.J.M. 277:953, 1967.

27. Weatherall, D.J., Edwards, J.A. and Donohoe, W.T.A. *Haemoglobin and Red Cell Enzyme Changes in Juvenile Myeloid Leukaemia.* Brit. Med. J. 1:679, 1968.

28. Beaven, G.H., Ellis, M.J. and White, J.C. *Studies on Human Foetal Haemoglobin: II. Foetal Haemoglobin Levels in Healthy Children and Adults and*

in Certain Haematological Disorders. Brit. J. Haemat. 6:201.

29. Rosa, J., Beuzard, Y., Brun, B. and Toulgoat, N. *Evidence for Various Types of Synthesis of Human γ Chains of Haemoglobin in Acquired Haematological Disorders*. Nature New Biology 233: 111, 1971.

30. Huisman, T.H.J., Schroeder, W.A., Bouver, N.G. Miller, A., Shelton, J.R., Shelton, J.B. and Apell, G. *Chemical Heterogeneity of Fetal Hemoglobin in Subjects with Sickle Cell Anemia, Homozygous Hb-C Disease, SC-Disease, and Various Combinations of Hemoglobin Variants*. Clin. Chim. Acta. 38:5, 1972.

31. Conley, C.L., Weatherall, D.J., Richardson, S.N., Shepard, M.K. and Charache, S. *Hereditary Persistance of Fetal Hemoglobin: A Study of 79 Affected Persons in 15 Negro Families in Baltimore*. Blood 21:261, 1963.

32. Wheeler, J.T. and Krevans, J.R. *The Homozygous State of Persistant Fetal Hemoglobin and the Interaction of Persistant Fetal Hemoglobin with Thalassemia*. Bull. Hopkins Hosp. 109:217, 1961.

33. Fessas, P. and Stomatoyannopoulos, G. *Hereditary Persistance of Fetal Hemoglobin in Greece. A Study and a Comparison*. Blood 24:223.

34. Huisman, T.H.J. and Schroeder, W.A. *New Aspects of the Structure, Function and Synthesis of Hemoglobins*. CRC Press, Cleveland, 1971.

35. Kendall, A.G., Ojwang, P.J., Schroeder, W.A. and Huisman, T.H.J. *Hemoglobin Kenja, The Product of a γ-β Fusion Gene: Studies of the Family*. Amer. J. Hum. Gen. 25:548, 1973.

36. Smith, D.H., Clegg, J.B., Weatherall, D.J. and Gilles, H.M. *Hereditary Persistance of Foetal Haemoglobin Associated with a γβ Fusion Variant Haemoglobin Kenja.* Nature New Biology 246:184, 1973.

37. Jacob, F. and Monod, J. *Genetic Regulatory Mechanisms in the Synthesis of Proteins.* J. Mol. Biol. 3:318, 1961.

38. Huisman, T.H.J., Schroeder, W.A., Efremov, G.D. Duma, H. , Mladenovski, B., Hyman, C.B., Rachmilewitz, E.A., Bouver, N., Miller, A., Brodie, A., Shelton, J.R., Shelton, J.B. and Apell, J. *The Present Status of the Heterogeneity of Fetal Hemoglobin in β-thalassemia: An Attempt to Unify Some Observations in Thalassemia and Related Conditions.* Ann. N.Y. Acad. 232:107, 1974.

39. Huehns, E.R., Dance, N., Beaven, G.H., Hecht, F. and Motulsky, A.G. *Human Embryonic Hemoglobins.* Cold Spring Harbor. Symp. Quart. Biol. 19:327, 1964.

40. Miyaji, T., Oba, Y., Yamamoto, K., Shibata, S., Iuchi, I. and Hamilton, H.B. *Hemoglobin Hijiyama: A New Fast-moving Hemoglobin in a Japanese Family.* Science 159:204, 1968.

41. Weatherall, D.J. *Hemoglobin J (Baltimore) Coexisting in a Family with Hemoglobin S.* Bull Hopkins Hosp. 114:1, 1964.

42. Swenson, R.T., Hill, R.L., Lehman, H. and Jim, R.T.S. *A Chemical Abnormality in Hemoglobin G from Chinese Individuals.* J. Biol. Chem. 237:1517, 1962.

43. Abramson, R.K., Rucknagel, D.L., Schreffler, D.C. and Saave, J.J. *Homozygous HbJ Tongariki: Evidence for only one Alpha Chain Structural Locus*

in Melanesians. Science 169:194, 1970.

44. Raper, A.B., Gammack, D.B., Huehns, E.R. and Shooter, E.M. *Four Haemoglobins in One Individual. A Study of the Genetic Interaction of HbG and HbC.* Brit. Med. J. 2:1257, 1960.

45. Weatherall, D.J., Sigler, A.T. and Baglioni, C. *Four Hemoglobins in Each of Three Brothers. Genetic and Biochemical Significance.* Bull. Hopkins Hosp. 111:143, 1962.

46. Wells, I.C. and Itano, H.A. *Ratio of Sickle-Cell Hemoglobin to Normal Hemoglobin in Sicklemics.* J. Biol. Chem. 188:65, 1951.

47. Nance, W.E. and Grove, J. *Genetic Determination of Phenotypic Variation in Sickle Cell Trait.* Science 177:716, 1972.

48. Neel, J.V., Wells, I.C. and Itano, H.A. *Familial Differences in the Proportion of Abnormal Haemoglobin Present in Sickle Cell Trait.* J. Clin. Invest. 30:1120, 1951.

49. Wasi, P., Pootrakul, S. and Na-Nakorn, S. *Hereditary Persistance of Foetal Haemoglobin in a Thai Family: The First Instance in the Mongol Race and in Association with Haemoglobin E.* Brit. J. Haemat. 14:501, 1968.

50. Feldman, R. and Rieder, R.F. *The Interaction of Hemoglobin E with β-thalassemia: A Study of Hemoglobin Synthesis in a Family of mixed Burmese and Iranian Origin.* Blood 42:783, 1973.

51. Frick, P.G., Hitzig, W.H. and Betke, K. *Hemoglobin Zurich I. A New Hemoglobin Anomaly Associated with Acute Hemolytic Episodes with Inclusion Bodies after Sulfonamide Therapy.* Blood 20:261, 1962.

52. Rieder, R.F., Zinkham, W.H. and Holtzmann, N.A. *Hemoglobin Zurich. Clinical, Chemical and Kinetic Studies.* Am. J. Med. 39:4, 1965.

53. Dickerman, J., Holtzmann, N.A. and Zinkham, W.H. *Hemoglobin Zurich. A Third Family Presenting with Hemolytic Reactions to Sulfonamides.* Am. J. Med. 55:638, 1973.

54. White, J.M. and Brain, M.C. *Defective Synthesis of an Unstable Haemoglobin: Haemoglobin Koln* (β^{98} val-met). Brit. J. Haemat. 18:195, 1970.

55. Halbrecht, I., Isaacs, W.A., Lehmann, H. and Ben-Porat, F. *Hemoglobin Hasharon* (α-47 *aspartic acid→histidine*). Israel J. Med. Sci. 3:827, 19

56. Charache, S., Mondzac, A.M., Gessner, V. and Gayle E.E. *Hemoglobin Hasharon* ($\alpha_2{}^{47\ his}{}_{(CD5)}\ \beta_2$): J. Clin. Invest. 48:834, 1969.

57. Schneider, R.G., Ueda, S., Alperin, J., Brimhall, B. and Jones, R.T. *Hemoglobin Sealy* ($\alpha_2{}^{47\ his}\beta$ *A New Variant in a Jewish Family.* Amer. J. Hum Gen. 20:151, 1968.

58. Crookston, J.H., Beale, D., Irvine, D. and Lehmann H. *A New Haemoglobin J. Toronto* (α5 alanine→aspartic acid). Nature 208:1059, 1965.

59. Clegg, J.B., Weatherall, D.J. and Milner, P.F. *Haemoglobin Constant Spring. A Chain Termination Mutant.* Nature 234:337, 1971.

60. Rieder, R.F., Wolf, D.J., Clegg, J.B. and Lee, S.L *Hemoglobin Bushwick, beta 74* (E18) *gly-val: An Unstable Hemoglobin Found in Extremely Small Amounts.* J. Clin. Invest. 53:65a, 1974.

61. Perrine, R.P., Brown, M.J., Clegg,J.B., Weatherall D.J. and May, A. *Benign Sickle-Cell Anaemia.* The Lancet 2:1163, 1972.

62. Wrightstone, R.N., Huisman, T.H.J. and Van Der Sar,A. *Qualitative and Quantitative Studies of Sickle Cell Hemoglobin in Homozygotes and Heterozygotes.* Clin. Chim. Act. 22:593, 1968.

63. DeSimone, J., Kleve, L., Longley, M.A. and Schaeffer, J. *Rapid Turnover of Newly Synthesized* β^S *Chains in Reticulocytes from Individuals with Sickle Cell Trait.* Biochem. Biophys. Res. Comm. 57:248, 1974.

64. Ranney, H.M. and Kono, P. *Studies of the Incorporation of* Fe^{59} *into Normal and Abnormal Hemoglobins.* J. Clin. Invest. 38:508, 1959.

65. Heywood, J.D., Karon, M. and Weissman, S. *Studies of in vitro Synthesis of Heterogenic Hemoglobins.* J. Clin. Invest. 43:2368, 1964.

66. Bank, A., O'Donnell, J.V. and Braverman, A.S. *Globin Chain Synthesis in Heterozygotes for* β *Chain Mutants.* J. Lab. Clin. Med. 76:616, 1970.

67. Heller, P., Yakulis, V.J., Epstein, R.B. and Friedland, S. *Variation in the Amount of Hemoglobin S in a Patient with Sickle Cell Trait and Megaloblastic Anemia.* Blood 21:479, 1965.

68. Wasi, P., Disthasonchan, P. and Na-Nakorn, S. *The Effect of Iron-deficiency on the Levels of Hemoglobins* A_2 *and* E. J. Lab. Clin. Med. 71:85, 1968.

69. Bradley, T.B., Jr., Wohl, R.L. and R. F. Rieder. *Hemoglobin Gun Hill: Deletion of Five Amino Acid Residues and Impaired Heme-globin Binding.* Science 157:1581, 1967.

70. Rieder, R.F. and Bradley, T.B., Jr. *Hemoglobin Gun Hill: An Unstable Protein Associated with Chronic Hemolysis.* Blood 32:355, 1968.

71. Rieder, R.F. *Synthesis of Hemoglobin Gun Hill: Increased Synthesis of the Heme-free* βGH *Globin Chain and Subunit Exchange with a Free* α-*chain pool*. J. Clin. Invest. 59:388, 1971.

72. Rieder, R.F. and James, G.W., III. *Imbalance in* α/β *Globin Synthesis Associated with a Hemoglobinopathy*. Blood 42:991, 1973.

73. Rieder, R.F. and James, G.W., III. *Imbalance in* α *and* β *Globin Synthesis Associated with a Hemoglobinopathy*. J. Clin. Invest. 54:948, 1974.

74. Rieder, R.F. *Translation of* β-*globin* mRNA *in* β-*thalassemia and the S and C Hemoglobinopathies*. J. Clin. Invest. 51:364, 1972.

75. Farace, M.G. and Bank, A. *Control of Human Hemoglobin Synthesis: Translation of Globin Chains in Heterozygotes with Hemoglobin Riverdale-Bronx*. Biochem. Biophys. Acta 312:591, 1973.

76. Rieder, R.F. Unpublished data.

77. Lang, A., Lehmann, H. and King-Lewis, P.A. *HbK Woolwich the Cause of a Thalassemia*. Nature 249:467, 1974.

78. Koler, R.D., Jones, R.T., Bigley, R.H., Litt, M., Lovrien, E., Brooks, R., Lahey, M.E. and Fowler, R. *Hemoglobin Casper:* β106 (G8) *Leu-pro. A Contemporary Mutation*. Amer. J. Med. 55:549, 1973.

79. Rieder, R.F. *Human Hemoglobin Stability and Instability: Molecular Mechanisms and Some Clinical Correlations*. Semin. in Hemat. 11:423, 197

80. Zalusky, R., Ross, J. and Katz, J.H. *Hb Riverdale-Bronx, An Unstable Hb. Differential Rates of Synthesis in the Heterozygote.* Blood 361:838, 1969.

81. Huehns, E.R. *The Unstable Hemoglobins.* Bull. Soc. Chim. Biol. 52:113, 1970.

82. White, J.M. and Dacie, J.V. *In vitro Protein Synthesis of Haemoglobin Hammersmith* CD1 *phe-ser.* Nature 225:939, 1970.

83. Steadman, J.H., Yates, A. and Huehns, E.R. *Idiopathic Heinz Body Anaemia: Hb Bristol (*β67 (E11) *val-asp).* Brit. J. Haemat. 18:435, 1970.

84. Cohen-Solal, M. and Labie, D. *A New Case of Hemoglobin Genova* $\alpha_2\beta_2^{28}$ (B10) *Leu→pro. Further Studies on the Mechanism of Instability and Defective Synthesis.* Biochim. Biophys. Acta 295: 67, 1973.

85. Honig, G.R., Mason, R.G., Vida, L.N. and Shamsudden, M. *Synthesis of Hemoglobin Abraham Lincoln (*β32 *leu-pro).* Blood 43:657, 1974.

86. Adams, J.G., III, Winter, W.P., Rucknagel, D.L. and Spencer, H.H. *Biosynthesis of Hemoglobin Ann Arbor: Evidence for Catabolic and Feedback Regulation.* Science 176:1427, 1972.

87. Lehmann, H. and Carrell, R.W. *Differences Between* α- *and* β-*chain Mutants of Human Haemoglobin and Between* α- *and* β-*thalassemia. Possible Duplication of the* α-*chain gene.* Brit. Med. J. 4:748, 1968.

88. Hollan, S.R., Szelenyi, J.G., Brimhall, B., Duerst, M., Jones, R.T., Koler, R.D. and Stocklen, Z. *Multiple Alpha Chain Loci for Human Haemoglobins: Hb J Buda and Hb G Pest.* Nature 235:47, 1972.

89. Luan Eng, L.-I., Ganesan, J., Clegg, J.B. and Weatherall, D.J. *Homozygous State for Hb Constant Spring. (Slow-moving Hb X Components).* Blood 43:251, 1974.

90. Rucknagel, D.L. and Winter, W.P. *Duplication of Structural Genes for Hemoglobin α and β Chains in Man.* Ann. N.Y. Acad. Sci. 241:80, 1974.

91. Weatherall, D.J., Clegg, J.B. and Naughton, M.A. *Globin Synthesis in Thalassemia: An in vitro Study.* Nature 208:1061, 1965.

92. Heywood, J.D., Karon, M. and Weissman, S. *Asymmetric Incorporation of Amino Acids into the Alpha and Beta Chains of Hemoglobin Synthesized in Thalassemia Reticulocytes.* J. Lab. Clin. Med. 66:476, 1965.

93. Bank, A. and Marks, P.A. *Excess Alpha Chain Synthesis Relative to Beta Chain Synthesis in Thalassaemia Major and Minor.* Nature 212:1198, 196

94. Clegg, J.B. and Weatherall, D.J. *Haemoglobin Synthesis in α-thalassaemia (Haemoglobin H Disease* Nature 215:1241.

95. Fessas, P ., Loukopoulos, D. and Kaltsoya, A. *Peptide Analysis of the Inclusions of Erythroid Cells in β-thalassemia.* Biochim. Biophys. Acta 124:430, 1966.

96. Rifkind, R.A. *Heinz-body Anemia: An Ultrastructural Study: II. Red Cell Sequestration and Destruction.* Blood 26:433, 1965.

97. Clegg, J.B., Weatherall, D.J., Na-Nakorn, S. and Wasi, P. *Haemoglobin Synthesis in β-thalassemi* Nature 220:664, 1968.

98. Nathan, D.G., Cividalli, G. and Lodish, H.F. *Translational Control of Hemoglobin Synthesis in Thalassemic Bone Marrow*. Ann. N.Y. Acad. Sciences 232:40, 1974.

99. Anderson, W.F. *Isolation and Translation of Messenger* RNA *from* β*thalassemia Red Cells*. Ann. N.Y. Acad. Sciences 232:15, 1974.

100. Benz, E.J., Jr. and Forget, B.G. *Defect in Messenger* RNA *for Human Hemoglobin Synthesis in Beta Thalassemia*. J. Clin. Invest. 50:2755, 1971.

101. Grossbard, E., Terada, M., Dow, L.W. and Bank, A. *Decreased* α *Globin Messenger* RNA *Activity Associated with Polyribosomes in* α*-thalassemia*. Nature New Biology 241:209, 1973.

102. Gambino, R., Kacian, D.L., Ramirez, F., Dow, L.W., Grossbard, E., Natta, C., Spiegelman, S., Marks, P.A. and Bank, A. *Decreased Globin Messenger* RNA *in Thalassemia by Hybridization and Biologic Activity Assays*. Ann. N.Y. Acad. Sci. 232:6, 1974.

103. Forget, B.G., Baltimore, D., Benz, E.J., Jr., Housman, D., Lebowitz, P., Marotta, C.A., McCaffrey, R.F., Skoultchi, A., Swerdlow, P.S., Verma, I.M. and Weissman, S. *Globin Messenger* RNA *in the Thalassemia Syndromes*. Ann. N.Y. Acad. Sci. 232:76, 1974.

104. Ottolenghi, S., Lanyon, W.G., Paul, J., Williamson, R., Weatherall, D.J., Clegg, J., Pritchard, J., Pootrakul, S., and Boon, W.H. *The Severe Form of* α *Thalassemia is Caused by a Haemoglobin Gene Deletion*. Nature 251:389, 1974.

105. Taylor, J.M., Dozy, A., Kan, Y.W., Varmus, H.E., Lie-Injo, L.E., Ganesin, J. and Todd, D. *Genetic Lesion in Homozygous* α *Thalassaemia (Hydrops Fetalis)*. Nature 251:392, 1974.

MECHANISMS OF HEMOGLOBIN S GELATION; STRUCTURAL RESTRICTIONS TO SUPRAMOLECULAR MODELS OF THE POLYMERIZATION OF Hb S

Dr. Ronald L. Nagel
Dr. Robert M. Bookchin

The last decade has been characterized by accelerated developments in the area of the molecular basis of sickling. The deformation of red cells containing Hb S when they are deprived of oxygen results from the formation of long Hb S polymers,which leads to gelation of the intracellular Hb. By electron microscopy, these polymers appear to have diameters of about 180 A^{o} and show a tendency to pack in a paracrystalline array with constant center-to-center distances (Fig. 1).

In considering the supramolecular architecture of these polymers, three basic questions are pertinent:

1. *What molecular conformation of the Hb molecule is required for polymerization?*
2. *Which areas on the surface of the Hb tetramer are involved in the protein-protein interactions or binding sites?*
3. *What type of bonds are involved in the binding?*

In the present paper we intend to review some old and some new data pertaining to these three questions. In several laboratories [1,2] optical and crystallographic studies have been employed in attempts to define the positions of some of the molecular axes and of the individual molecules in the polymer and thus to determine the pattern of molecular stacking. Depending upon the precision of such studies, the general regions of intermolecular contacts may or may not be defined. Our laboratory, on the other hand, has approached these questions through studies of the effects on gelation and sickling of specific modifications of the Hb S tetramer or its environment, using other Hb mutants, as well as chemical modifications and ligand hybrids of Hb S. These two approaches are not in conflict and may very well prove to be complementary.

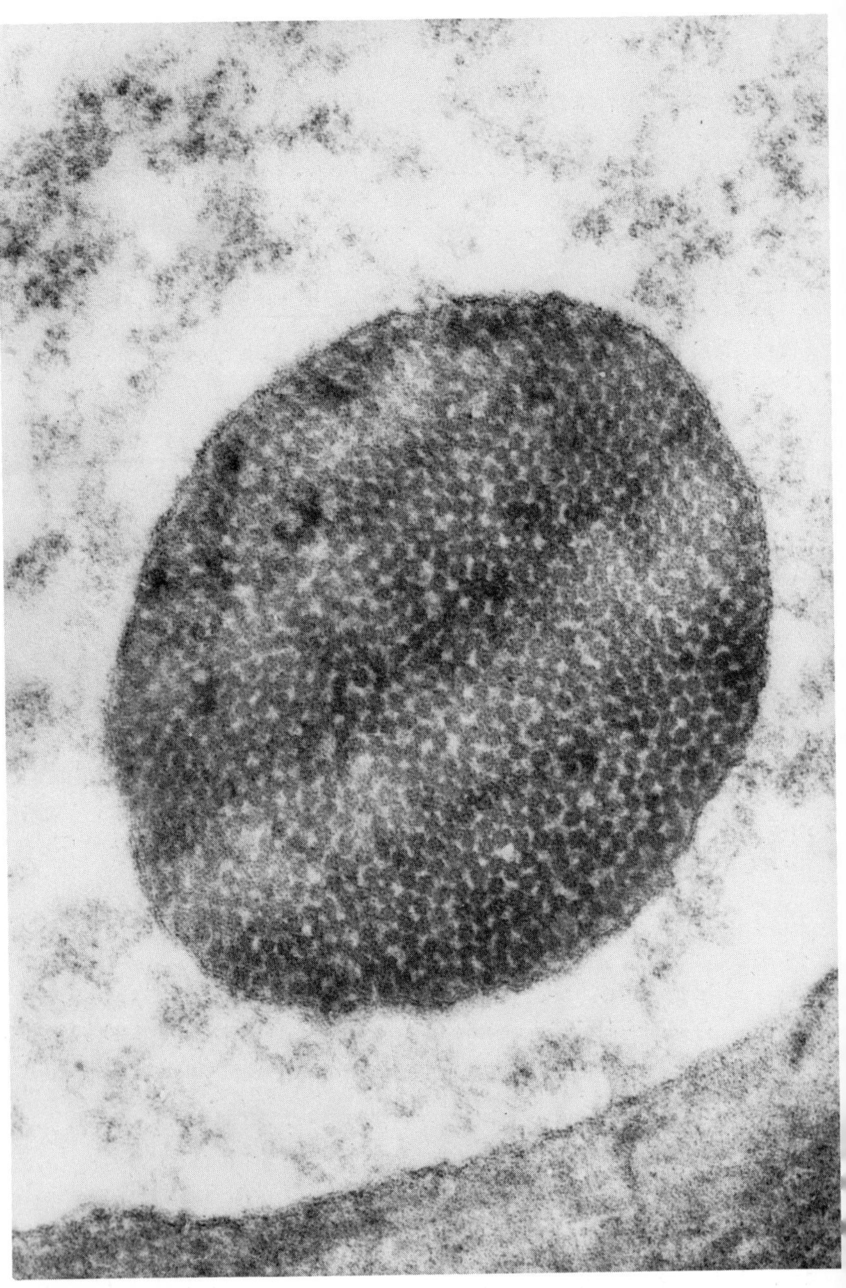

Fig. 1. Electron micrograph of cross-section of a prot[o]plasmic prolongation of a sickled (SS) red cell in the deoxy state. The dots are cross-sections of microtubul[es]. Occasional paracrystalline packing is seen in areas whe[re] the center-to-center distance between fibers is constan[t]. x 75,000. (Courtesy of Isabel Tellez-Nagel, M.D.).

Let us now consider the three questions posed:

1. What Hb S conformer favors polymerization?

The best evidence that the T conformer (equated by Perutz[3] to the fully deoxygenated conformation of hemoglobin) is the preferred form of Hb S for polymerization stems from the work of Bookchin and Nagel on mixed liganded hybrids[4]. The minimum gelling concentration (MGC) of $\alpha_2\beta_2^{S*}$ (in which * refers to CN met form and the companion subunits are deoxy) are notably indistinguishable: 33.5 gm/dl. This suggests that the r → t (tertiary) structural changes induced by the absence of the ligand in the mutant β chain alone is *not* sufficient to provide an optimal conformational change for maximal interaction. It appears, rather, that the quaternary change R → T is indispensable and, as reflected in the gelling behavior of Hb S, is equivalent for both half-liganded hybrids. It should be noted that other evidence suggests that such mixed liganded hybrids indeed have a deoxy-like quaternary conformation (although apparently somewhat different from fully deoxy Hb A).

2. *What are the binding areas?*

It appears likely that the substitution directly determines at least one of the binding sites (β6Val - determined site). The most direct evidence for this is that nitrogen mustard inhibits gelling of Hb S by modifying H is 2β, which presumably alters this primary binding site [5].

The inhibition of gelation by β^{73Asn} in Hb C_{Harlem} ($\alpha_2\beta_2$ $^{6Val,\ 73Asn}$) and in mixtures of Hb Korle Bu ($\alpha_2\beta_2$ ^{73Asn}) with Hb S strongly suggests that β^{73} residue is involved in an area of interaction. Furthermore, the inhibitory effect of β^{73Asn} substitution is exaggerated at low ionic strength; under these conditions, Hb S gels more readily (see below) while Hb C Harlem fails to gel. This raises the possibility that an electrostatic bond involving the -COO- of the normal residue, β^{73Asp}, is important in an area of intermolecular contact in the polymerization of deoxy Hb S[6,7].

But the most striking and informative finding is that admixture of Hb A to Hb C_{Harlem} corrects the inhibition of β^{73Asn} and renders the mixture indistinguishable from Hb S/Hb A[6]. These results, interpreted in the context of hybrid ($\alpha_2\beta^A\beta^C$ Harlem) formation, suggest that the role of each β chain in the tetramer is different and distinct. When β^{73} coexists with β6Val in the same chain, and the other β chain is normal, the interaction is normal. When one β chain contains β6Val substitution and the other the $\beta^{73\ Asn}$ substitution (Hb Korle Bu/Hb S or Hb C $_{Harlem}$ alone) the interactions are diminished.

The question follows: *Is the* β6Val *area active in one chain and inactive in the other during polymerization?* The answer has been provided by MGC determinations on mixtures of Hb S with mutants having substitutions in the β6Val area, such as Hb Leiden ($\alpha_2\beta_2$ Del 6 or 7), Hb G Makassar ($\alpha_2\beta_2{}^{2Ala}$) and Hb Deer Lodge ($\alpha_2\beta_2{}^{2Arg}$). As showin in Table 1, the MGC of these mixtures is indistinguishable from Hb S/Hb A, all of which gel at 32 gm/dl.

TABLE 1. *MINIMUM GELLING CONCENTRATIONS OF MIXTURES OF Hb S WITH OTHER MUTANTS OF THE NH_2-TERMINAL OF THE β CHAIN**

	MGC g/dl
40% Hb S + 60% Hb A	32
40% Hb S + 60% Hb Leiden ($\alpha_2\beta_2{}^{6Glu\rightarrow 0}$)	32
40% Hb S + 60% Hb Makassar ($\alpha_2\beta_2$6Glu→Ala)	32
40% Hb S + 60% Hb Deer Lodge ($\alpha_2\beta_2{}^{2His\rightarrow Arg}$)	32

*Hemoglobin variants isolated by column chromatography and found to contain less than 5% met hemoglobin by spectrophotometry. MGC determined at 22°, 0.15M phosphate buffer, pH 7.35.

In view of the likelihood that the companion hemoglobins copolymerize with Hb S as symmetrical hybrids, it can be concluded that the second β chain (S or non-S) participates in the polymer with interactions that do not involve the β6Val area. This notion is strengthened by the same finding in mixtures of Hb S with Hb A alkylated with nitrogen mustard (a reagent that inhibits polymerization of deoxy Hb S by modifying His 2β)[5].

Other residues have been implicated in the polymerization of Hb S. The increased participation in gelation with deoxy Hb S reported for Hb D Los Angeles ($\alpha_2\beta_2$ $^{121\ Glu \rightarrow Gln}$)[8] and perhaps even greater participation of Hb O_{Arab} ($\alpha_2\beta_2$$^{121\ Glu \rightarrow Lys}$)[9] is an example of the converse situation, in which the elimination of an anionic side chain ($Glu^- \rightarrow Gln$) improves interaction, and introduction of a cationic side chain ($Glu^- \rightarrow Lys^+$) improves it further. The location of β^{121}(GH4) on the hemoglobin molecule is not far from β^{73} (E17) so that it is conceivable that one region of contact is involved.

Thus far almost all examples of variations in participation of non-S hemoglobins involve β chain substitutions. The only instance in which an α chain substitution was shown to affect sickling interactions was in Hb Memphis/S in which $\alpha^{23 Glu \rightarrow Gln}$ appeared to result in decreased interactions and a milder clinical course[10].

One region that can be excluded from participation in the binding sites is that of β73Cys. When p-hydroximercuribenzoate is used to block this residue (with quite a bulky side chain) no effect is observed in the gelling of Hb S, Hb C_{Harlem} and sickle trait blood (Table 2).

Another interesting aspect relating to the binding sites in Hb S polymerization concerns the effect of 2,3 diphosphoglycerate (2,3 DPG) on this phenomenon. This co-factor has been shown to promote red cell sickling and aggregation of deoxy Hb S solutions. Elevation of 2,3 DPG was found by Paniker et al.[11] to increase the viscosity of fully deoxygenated solutions of Hb S. Briehl and Ewart[12], using ultracentrifugal techniques, have demonstrated that addition of 2,3 DPG to "stripped" Hb S in non-phosphate buffers lowers the minimum gelling concentration (MGC) of the deoxy Hb.

TABLE 2. *EFFECT OF pMB REACTED β93 Cys ON MGC OF Hb S AND Hb* C_{Harlem}*

	MGC gm/dl
Hb S	23.8
Hb S-pMB	24.2
Hb C_H	36.2
Hb C_H-pMB	36.2
Hb SA	32.1
Hb SA-pMB	33.2

*Hemoglobin solutions were exposed to a 2.5 molar excess (per mole tetramer) of p-hydroximercuribenzoate (pMB) and passed through a Sephadex G-25 column, after which titration showed no reactive -SH groups. MGC's were determined at 22° in 0.15M phosphate buffer, pH7.35.

By measuring sickling as a function of saturation of red cell Hb with O_2 in cells in which 2,3 DPG had been artificially raised or lowered in vitro, Jensen et al[13] showed that the enchancement of sickling by 2,3 DPG is greater than that due to the lowered oxygen affinity.

There are at least two mechanisms by which 2,3 DPG could promote gelation of Hb S: *1.) by stabilizing the deoxy (T) conformation of the tetramer, which appear to be the preferred form of polymerization, and 2.) by induction of tertiary conformational changes in regions of the molecule which are involved in intermolecular binding.* These two mechanisms are not mutually exclusive, but the possible roles of each could not be distinguished by previous studies.

We have designed experiments to help resolve these possible mechanisms by studying the effect of 2,3 DPG on gelation of deoxy Hb S under conditions in which the R-T equilibrium is not further altered by addition of

2,3 DPG, and by observing the effects on gelation of altering the R-T equilibrium in the absence of 2,3 DPG.

The effects of 2,3 DPG on the MGC of "stripped" deoxy Hb S are shown in Table 3.

TABLE 3. *MINIMUM GELLING CONCENTRATION OF "STRIPPED" Hb S IN THE ABSENCE AND PRESENCE OF 2,3 DIPHOSPHO-GLYCERATE.*

(2,3 DPG)/(Hb)	MGC g/dl
0	23.5
5:1	20.2
10:1	20.4

The Hb S solutions were "stripped" of inorganic and organic phosphates by dialysis for 16 hrs. against 0.1M NaCl, using No. 20 cellulose casing (Union Carbide Co.) which had been previously stretched. Buffer: 0.05M bis-Tris, pH 7.35, with 0.1M NaCl. Temperature: 22°C.

These findings, which show that 2,3 DPG enhances gelation of deoxy Hb S, are consistent with the viscosity observations of Paniker et al.[11] and confirm the ultracentrifugal studies of Briehl and Ewart[12].

The data in Fig.2 show the effect of increasing amounts of 2,3 DPG on the MGC of deoxy Hb S which had previously been dialyzed against 0.15M K phosphate buffer, pH 7.35. Note that in the absence of 2,3 DPG, the MGC of Hb S in the 0.15M phosphate buffer is the same as it is in 0.05M bis-Tris, pH 7.35 with 0.1M NaCl (between 23 and 24 gm Hb/100 ml). With addition of 2,3 DPG, the MGC falls to about 20 gm Hb/100 ml, with the maximum effect at concentrations of 8 to 10 moles 2,3 DPG per mole Hb tetramer. Since the dissociation contant for the reaction between Hb and 2,3 DPG at this pH is about 4×10^{-5}M [8], it appears that the maximal effect of 2,3 DPG on the MGC occurs at concentrations at which the Hb would be saturated with the organic phosphate.

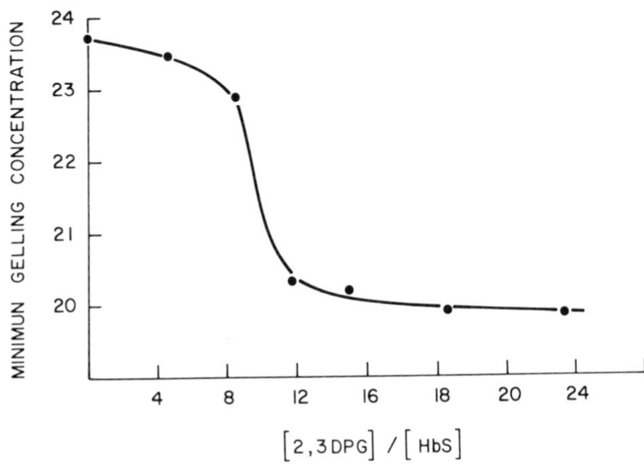

Fig. 2. The effect of increasing amounts of 2,3 DPG on the minimum gelling concentration of deoxy Hb S. Abscissa: molar ratio of 2,3 DPG per hemoglobin tetramer. Samples dialyzed against 0.15M K phosphate, pH 7.35. Temperature 22°C.

In Fig. 3 it is shown that the oxygen affinity of Hb in 0.15M K phosphate pH 7.35 is considerably lower than it is in 0.05M bis-Tris with 0.1M NaCl, at the same pH; but in the presence of 0.15M phosphate, addition of a 10 molar excess of 2,3 DPG per mole Hb has no further effect on the oxygen affinity of Hb.

Let us now consider the implications of these findings on the mechanism by which 2,3 DPG facilitates gelation and sickling. If we first compare the behavior of Hb in 0.15M phosphate buffer and in 0.05M bis-Tris with 0.1M NaCl, in the absence of 2,3 DPG, it is clear that the R-T equilibrium is shifted more towards the T form in the presence of phosphate. In other words, phosphate tends to stabilize the deoxy (T) conformation. Nevertheless, the MGC of fully deoxy Hb S is equivalent in both buffered media. This suggests that <u>when Hb S is fully deoxygenated</u> the effect of substances which "stabilize the deoxy conformation" (simply in terms of altering the oxygen affinity and R-T equilibrium) have no significant effect on the tendency to polymerize.

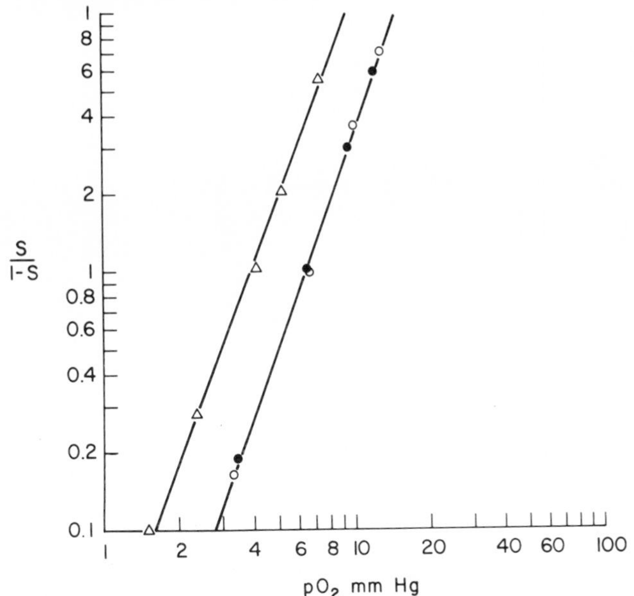

Fig. 3. Oxygen dissociation curve of Hb S plotted according to the logarithmic form of Hill's equation. S=fractional saturation. pO_2=partial pressure of oxygen in mm of mercury. -Δ- Hb S, in 0.05M bis-Tris, 0.1M NaCl, pH 7.22. -O- Hb S, 0.15M K phosphate, pH 7.35 and -●- Hb S, 0.15M K phosphate + 10 molar excess of 2,3 DPG, pH 7.35. Temperature 22°C.

Now we look at the effect of addition of 2,3 DPG in the presence of 0.15M phosphate, we see that there is no further effect on the oxygen affinity (and thus no alteration of the R-T equilibrium), but there is a considerable increase in the tendency of deoxy Hb S to polymerize: the MGC is lowered from 23.7 to 20 gm Hb/ 100 ml. In collaboration with Dr. Peter R.B. Caldwell of Columbia University, we have furthermore demonstrated that the same pattern is observed in 0.5M phosphate buffer. In this media, the addition of 2,3 DPG produces no further decrease in the oxygen affinity of highly concentrated Hb solutions, but results in a significant decrease in the MGC.

Arnone [14] has demonstrated by X-ray crystallograph that 2,3 DPG binds deoxy Hb in the central cavity by salt-bridge linkages to three paired β chain residues (valines NA1, histidines NA2 and histidines H21) and to a single β lysine residue (lysine EF6). This accounts for the 1:1 stoichiometry of the binding 2,3 DPG to Hb, the preferential binding to deoxy Hb, and the shift in the R-T equilibrium (lowered oxygen affinity). To achieve the oxy (R) state, the β chains must rotate about 7Å towards each other; by impairing this change, 2,3 DPG stabilizes the deoxy (T) conformation.

Apart from this quaternary structural effect, however, Arnone has shown that binding of 2,3 DPG produces tertiary structural alterations in both β chains: the NA and initial A helical segments of the β chains are 2 to 3Å closer together. These alterations involve the region of the substitution in Hb S: Val NA3 (β6). The experiments described above indicate that the mechanism by which 2,3 DPG promotes gelation of fully deoxygenated Hb S is independent from its effect on the R-T equilibrium (and "stabilization" of the deoxy (T) form), and suggest that the additional structural alterations in the Hb tetramer induced by the binding of 2,3 DPG (such as those described by Arnone), which are independent of the R-T equilibrium, are responsible for these effects. Such a mechanism is also likely to be operative in partly deoxygenated erythrocytes.

It is possible that the other effect of 2,3 DPG, stabilization of the T state, could also play a role in its oxygen affinity-independent action of promoting sickling at intermediate states of oxygenation. However, as a result of cooperativity, the concentration of partially oxygenated molecules is likely to be quite low, so that the potential contribution of this second effect is probably minimal. *3.) What type of bonds stabilize the polymer?*

Observations that the gel of deoxy Hb S liquifies at low temperature or high pressure have been cited in favor of an important role for hydrophobic interactions in the polymerization of Hb S. Nevertheless, there has been no systematic study of the extent and details of these interactions. Recently, Dr. Danek Elbaum has examined this aspect of Hb S interaction in our laboratory[15]. In the presence of 0.15M K phosphate, pH 7.35, 22°, addition of 0.1M urea, methylurea, ethylurea, propylurea and butylurea raised the MGC from 23-24 gm Hb/dl to 25.6, 28.0, 31.7, 33.4 and 33.8 gm/dl, respectively. An analogous trend was found upon addition of 0.2M alkylureas. Thus, with progressive increase in the length of the hydrocarbon chain of the alkylureas, there is progressive inhibition of gelation of deoxy Hb S. As judged by ORD studies, these concentrations of alkylureas produce no alteration of the secondary structure of Hb S. Furthermore, 0.1M ethylurea or propylurea have no effects on the oxygen affinity or cooperativity of normal Hb, (although they do raise the oxygen affinity of whole blood from patients with sickle cell anemia, presumably by interfering with the gelation process). These findings support the notion that hydrophobic interactions indeed play a role in the stabilization of the polymer and open a methodological approach to the quantitative study of this aspect of the process.

But the hydrophobic interactions are not the only non-covalent bonds involved in these protein-protein interactions. Our findings that exhaustively dialyzed solutions of Hb S gel at much lower concentration than they do in the presence of salts suggests that electrostatic bonds between the molecules are also involved in the polymerization; accordingly, the increase in the gelling point with increments in ionic strength (over the range tested) may result from the shielding of surface charges of the protein in molecules by dissolved electrolytes.

Finally, the effect of D_2O on the MGC of Hb S is quite remarkable. As it can be seen in Table 4, the replacement of exchangeable hydrogen by deuterium significantly enhances the polymerizing tendencies of deoxy Hb S. This enhancement could be the result of an increase in the strength of hydrophobic interactions, hydrogen bonds, or both. In addition, this effect is additive with the effect of low ionic strength, resulting in the lowest MGC values that we have observed with this method.

TABLE 4. *EFFECT OF D_2O ON THE MGC OF DEOXY HbS**

0.15 M PO_4, pH 7.35	23.5
" in D_2O	18.7
Dialyzed against H_2O	14.0
" in D_2O	9.5

*D_2O exchange was performed in Diaflo 8MCMicro-Ultrafiltration System (Amicon Corp.).

4. *Molecular Restrictions:*

If we assume that non S hemoglobin copolymerize with Hb S by forming symmetrical hybrid tetramers ($\alpha_2\beta^S\beta^X$), the following conclusions can be drawn:

1.) *The quaternary deoxy conformer (and not intrachain t $\rightleftarrows$ r changes) seems to be a prerequisite for the polymerization of Hb S.*

2.) *There is more than one intermolecular contact area for each tetramer.*

3.) *Each of the two β chains of a tetramer provides a different region of contact in the polymer. One of the β chains contributes the β6 Val region but its β73 region is not in a contact area. For the other β chain, the β73 region is involved in an intermolecular contact, but β6 Val is not.*

4.) *The displacement of the two β6 Val regions of the tetramer 2 Å closer to each other upon binding 2,3 DPG, (as demonstrated by Arnone), favors polymerization of deoxy Hb S.*

5.) *The region of β93 Cysteine in Hb S and Hb C_{Harlem} is not involved in any binding sites.*

6.) *Both hydrophobic and electrostatic interactions (and possibly also hydrogen binding) are involved in the stabilization of Hb S polymers.*

5. *Model Building:*

At this point we may ask whether it is possible to construct a molecular model of the microtubular polymer which is in accordance with the above restrictions as well as with the electron microscopic and other optical (1,2) findings? The latter include the following restrictions:

a.) *The Hb S molecules generate the microtubule by stacking in discs of six tetramers each*[1].

b.) *The x* ($\alpha_1\beta_1$ *pseudo-dyad) axis of the tetramer is placed within a small angle (less than 22°) of the fiber axis*[2].

It can be shown (Fig.4) that the Hb molecules can be stacked so as to comply with the restrictions described in paragraph 4.

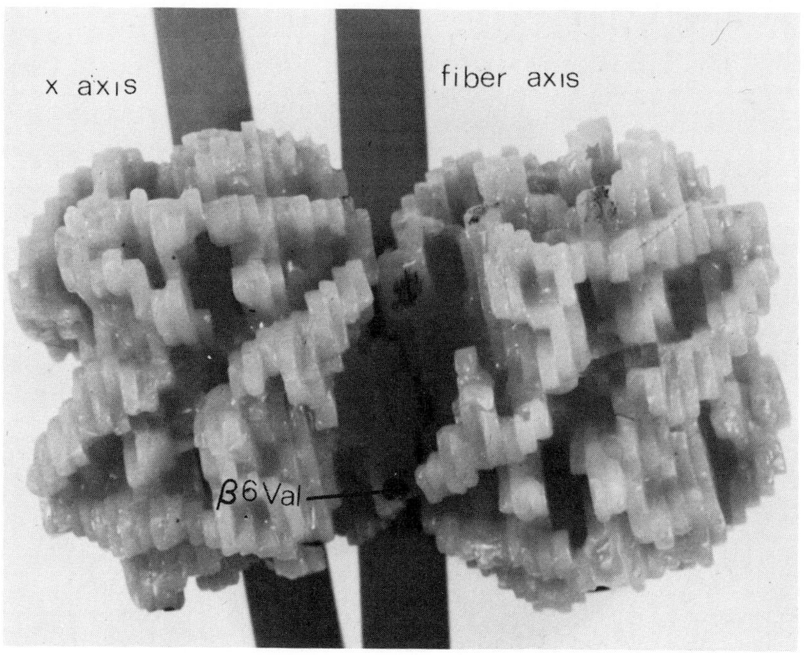

Fig. 4. Model building with plastic models based on the available electron density maps of deoxy hemoglobin 5 Å resolution. Fiber axis, x axis and β6Val site are identified. The dyad (y) axis is tangential to the fiber axis.

This is achieved by placing the dyad (y) axis of symmetry tangential and the z axis radial to the fiber or microtubule, accommodating only one of the β6 Val sites in lateral interactions. Viewing this packing from the direction of the fiber axis, as in Fig. 5, one can readily see that the mutations known to modify polymerization are indeed in a position to interact at the disc-disc interfaces (vertically).

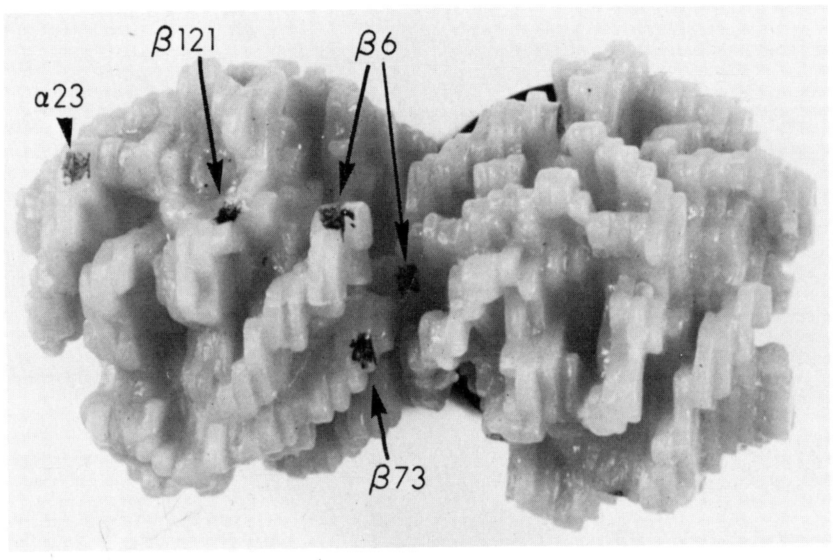

Fig. 5. Model of the packing illustrated in Fig. 4, but now observed from the fiber axis.

A word of caution is in order: Model building is only a rough approximation to reality and in this case is based on limited data. In addition, the fact that a particular model fits the data does not mean that it is the correct solution. It would seem highly unlikely that an accurate model could be constructed by the use of high resolution coordinates derived from studies of Hb A. No solid information exists that the conformation of Hb S in the deoxy form (or for that matter in the oxy form) is identical with that of Hb A. Preliminary nuclear magnetic resonance studies of Ho and associates[16], and the increased precipitability of oxy Hb S with mechanical agitation[17] suggests that there may, in fact, be considered conformational differences between hemoglobins S and A. Our model building utilizes only low resolution (5Å) information.

The final solution of this problem will come when the supramolecular and molecular data are brought together by further experimentation.

ACKNOWLEDGEMENTS

This publication was made possible by the following supportive Grants: NHLI-2-2920, NIH 15053, AM13430, AM 12597 and 5-PO-1-GM-19100.

REFERENCES

1. Finch, J.T., Perutz, M.F. and Bertles, J.F. Proc. Nat. Acad. Sci. USA 70:718, 1973.

2. Hofrichter, J., Hendricker, D.G. and Eaton, W.A. Proc. Nat. Acad. Sci. 70:3604, 1973.

3. Perutz, M.F. Nature (Lond.) 228:726, 1970.

4. Bookchin, R.M. and Nagel, R.L. J. Mol. Bio. 60:263, 1971.

5. Roth, E.F., Jr., Nagel, R.L. and Bookchin, R.M. Clin. Res. 20:565, 1973.

6. Bookchin, R.M., Nagel, R.L. and Ranney, H.M. J. Biol. Chem., 242:248, 1967.

7. Bookchin, R.M., Nagel, R.L. and Ranney, H.M. Biochim. Biophys. Acta 221:373, 1970.

8. Charache, S., Conley, C.L., Waugh, D.F. J. Clin. Invest. 46:1795, 1967.

9. Milner, P.F., Miller, C., Grey, R., Seakins, M., De-Jong, W.W. and Went, L.N. N. Engl. Med. 283:1417, 1970.

10. Kraus, L.M., Miyaji, T., luchi, J. and Kraus, A.P. Biochemistry 5:3701, 1966.

11. Paniker, N.V., Ben-Bassat, I. and Beutler, E. J. Lab. Clin. Med. 80:282, 1972.

12. Briehl, R.W. and Ewert, S. J. Mol. Biol. 80:445, 1973.

13. Jensen, M., Bunn, H.F., Halikas, G., Kan, Y.W. and Nathan, D.G. J. Clin. Invest. 52:2542, 1973.

14. Arnone, A. Nature 237:146, 1972.

15. Elbaum, D., Nagel, R.L., Bookchin, R.M. and Herskovits, T.T. Proc. U.S. Nat. Acad. Sci. (in press).

16. Ho, C. and Fung, L. Proceedings of the First National Symposium on Sickle Cell Anemia. Washington, 1974.

17. Asakura, T., Ohnishi, T., Friedman, S. and Schwartz E. Proc. U.S. Nat. Acad. Sci. 71:1594, 1974.

PATHOGENESIS OF SICKLE CELL DISEASE

John F. Bertles, M.D.

The major purpose of this section of the Symposium is to describe the manner in which basic defects in the erythrocytes of patients with sickle cell anemia (Hb SS disease) might produce the ultimate pathologic picture. It should be emphasized that we are talking about a "small vessel" disease. Diggs (1973) has recently provided us with a comprehensive description of the pathology of sickle syndromes; and "it is apparent that the gradual attrition suffered by patients with this affliction derives from luminal occlusion of small vessels by Hb SS erythrocytes in various stages of reversible and irreversible deformation." On physical examination, this entrapment of Hb SS erythrocytes in small vessels is most obvious in the terminal blood vessels of the bulbar conjunctiva (Fig. 1).

The fact that erythrocytes must navigate through capillary channels frequently narrower than the red cells themselves is one of the most perilous aspects of the sickle syndromes. During the time that any erythrocyte makes its round trips from heart through capillary beds and back to the heart, a mandatory capability is that of deformability. The real job of red cells is performed in the microcirculation, and a normal erythrocyte (Hb AA) must make this round trip many times. Figure 2 sketches the difficulties that a red cell encounters when it must pass through a capillary of very narrow dimensions. It is intuitively apparent that the ability to squeeze through this passage is permitted by the large ratio of surface area to volume characteristic of normal red cells. Thus the large surface area permits hemoglobin to flow in the cell during passage in such a way that, sausage-like, the cell can navigate successfully.

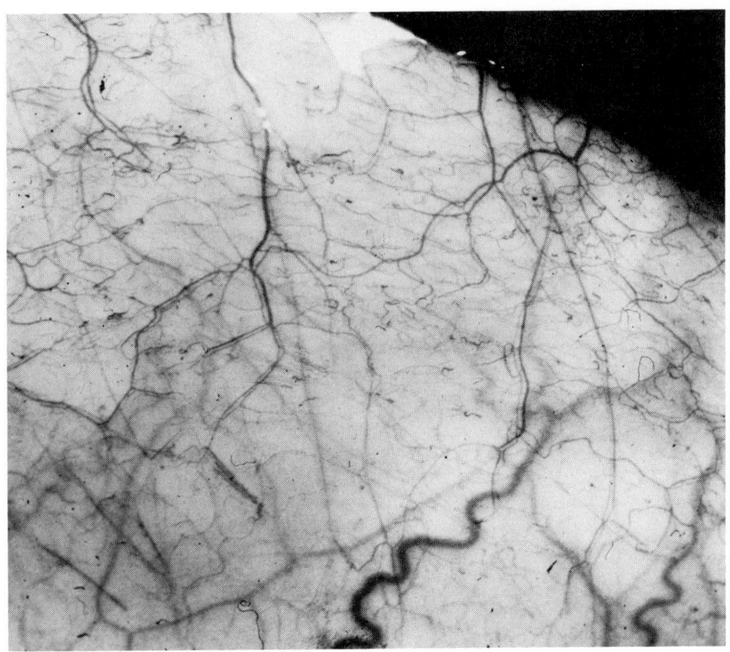

Fig. 1. Photograph of bulbar conjunctiva of an Hb SS patient. Sacculations in terminal vessels are caused by aggregations of sickled erythrocytes. From Diggs (1973).

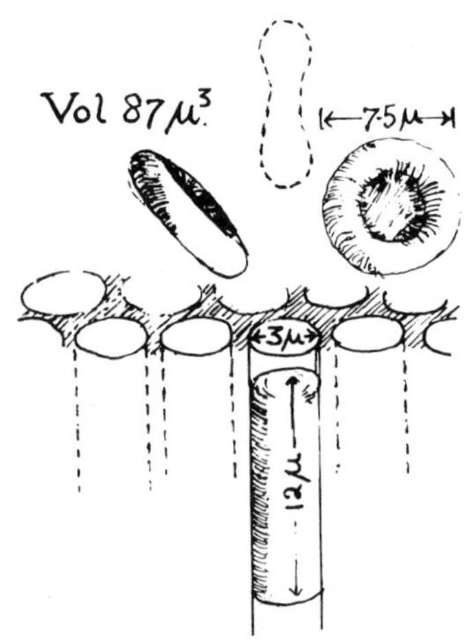

Fig. 2. Schematic representation of a normal erythrocyte and its need to deform in order to pass through a narrow-bore capillary. From Burton (1966).

And obviously this extremely close proximity to the capillary wall permits maximal exposure of the red cell surface to the area where gas diffusion must take place, both in the lungs and in the peripheral tissues. In any discussion of pathogenesis in the sickle syndromes, it cannot be too strongly emphasized that lack of red cell deformability is a crucial problem. Reasons for this will become apparent in a moment. Of course the sickle syndromes do not hold a monopoly on lack of red cell deformability. There are numerous diseases in man in which erythrocytes have difficulty traversing the microcirculation: altered red cell membranes, altered cell contents, and altered cell shape all lead to similar difficulties, but in none of these other diseases of man are the results of lack of deformability so traumatic as Hb SS disease.

A considerable amount of information can be gathered from simple examination of a peripheral blood smear from an Hb SS patient. Before describing the significance of the proportion of permanently deformed cells in the peripheral blood, I wish to describe here, as an illustration of how complicated the pathogenesis of sickle syndromes may become, the clinical course of a patient recently seen by us (Cameron et al, 1971). The patient was a 22 year old woman with Hb SC disease. Cardiac catheterization demonstrated severe mitral stenosis and insufficiency of both mitral and aortic valves. Cardiac decompensation, increasingly difficult to control, seemed to be an absolute indication for surgical valve replacement, but we were of course reluctant to introduce the added damage that artificial valves might cause to her already compromised red cells. The operation became mandatory, and the risk of sickling at operation was diminished by a 70% partial exchange transfusion with normal erythrocytes accomplished at the time of cardiac bypass. Despite the development of marked red cell fragmentation, known to be associated with the presence of ball valve prostheses, the patient did well after the operation and her red cell life span was not changed. However, approximately one year after the operation, her hemoglobin level began to drop and it was noted that she demonstrated marked macrocytosis in the peripheral blood. She had indeed developed severe folic acid deficiency, well known to be associated with the chronic hemolytic states. This vignette is intended to emphasize that, while contemplating the pathogenesis of the sickle syndromes, one must not ignore the possibility of other pathology and the ever present possibility of complications of the disease itself.

The bizarre silhouettes assumed by Hb SS erythrocytes when partially or totally deoxygenated are well known to most clinicians. Recently, however, considerable information has been gathered by examining those cells in the peripheral blood of Hb SS patients that are permanently deformed even when fully oxygenated. Figure 3 shows the *oxygenated* peripheral blood of an Hb SS patient.

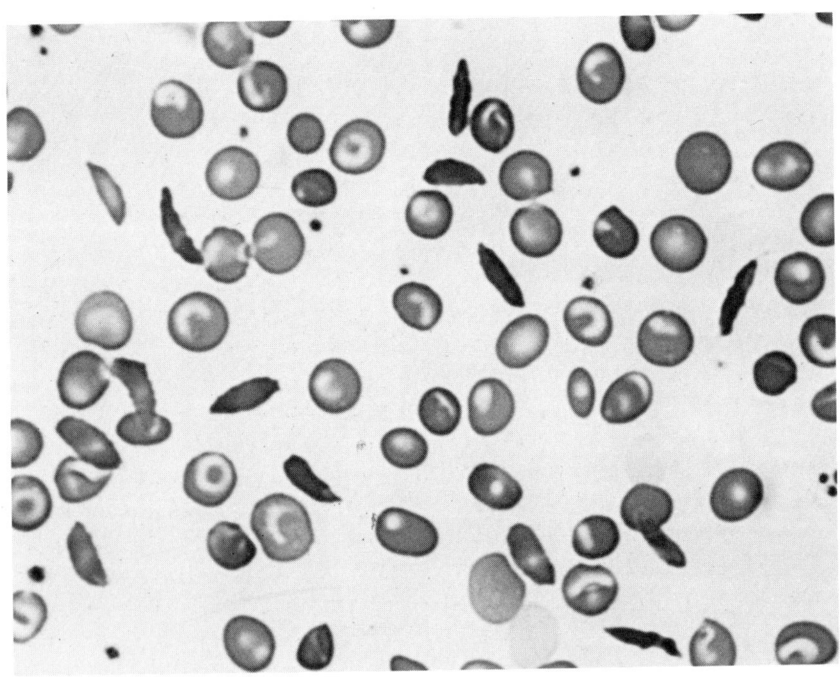

Fig. 3. Photomicrograph of the oxygenated peripheral blood of an Hb SS patient. Numerous irreversibly "sickled" cells (ISC), actually permanently deformed and not truly sickled, are apparent. From Bertles, 1973

Several pathologic mechanisms may be responsible for the development of these irreversibly deformed erythrocytes, often called irreversibly "sickled" cells (ISC), ranging from the morphologically obvious membrane damage suffered by Hb SS erythrocytes during sickle-unsickle cycles (Jensen and Klug, 1973) to the more subtle metabolic alterations proposed by Eaton and co-workers (1973) and Jensen and co-workers (1973). These latter investigations suggest that Hb SS erythrocytes are excessively permeable to calcium, and that somehow the attachment of calcium to the endoface of the erythrocyte generates the irreversible deformation characteristic of ISC. Thus when an Hb SS erythrocyte emerges from the bone marrow it is confronted by several ominous options: removal from the circulation as a reversibly deformable erythrocyte, or development into an irreversibly deformed cell which has been shown to have a preferentially shortened life span (Bertles and Milner, 1968). It must be emphasized that the morphologically obvious irreversibly deformed erythrocyte is only the end point in what must be the gradual development of abnormalities in Hb SS erythrocytes during their characteristically shortened life span. Although ISC are characterized by a greatly increased MCHC (Bertles and Milner, 1968; Chien et al., 1970; Seakins et al., 1973), a gradual increase in MCHC appears to occur in reversibly deformable Hb SS erythrocytes as they age. Recently a relationship has been drawn between the well-known right-shift of the oxygen saturation curve of Hb SS blood to this increase in MCHC (Seakins et al., 1973). Indeed, the higher the MCHC in Hb SS erythrocytes separated according to density by ultracentrifugation, the further is the saturation curve shifted to the right. The implication of the saturation curve shift, of course, is that high MCHC erythrocytes would, therefore, sickle more readily than normal MCHC Hb SS erythrocytes at any given PO_2. Hence the ISC is a triple hazard in the circulation: it appears that the cell membrane, somehow damaged, is deformed and stiff; the MCHC is so high that the internal viscosity of the cell must be an absolute deterrent to the passage of the cell through the microcirculation (Chien et al., 1970); and the oxygen saturation is dangerously shifted to the right. Note, in Figure 4, that the increase in viscosity as hemoglobin concentration rises is not a function of the type of hemoglobin present (that is, Hb S compared with Hb A), but is only a function of the concentration of hemoglobin.

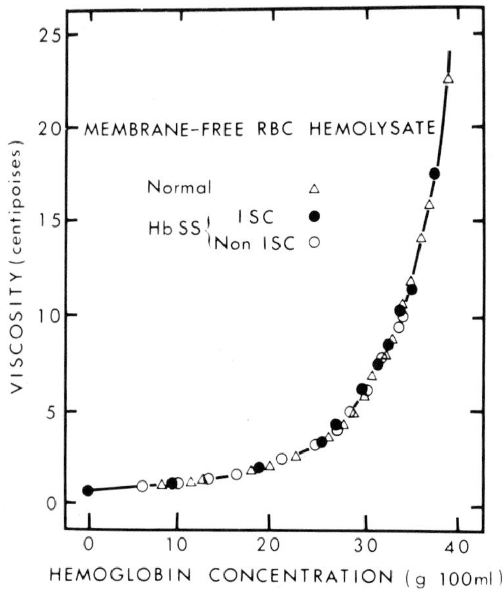

Fig. 4. Relationship between hemoglobin concentration and viscosity in oxygenated cell-free solutions. Hb S and Hb A fall on the same curve. From Chien et al.,1970

As some of these ISC have an MCHC as high as 45 gm/ 100 ml, it is obvious that these are indeed very sick cells.

Further generalizations can be made concerning the clinical status of an Hb SS patient and the proportion of his peripheral red cells made up by these irreversibly deformed erythrocytes. For example, work by others has shown that the degree of shortening of an Hb SS patient's red cell survival time (as measured as ^{51}Cr T½) is directly related to the proportion of ISC in the peripheral blood. Nevertheless, all of us in clinical hematology have seen any number of Hb SS patients who do quite well despite a large number of permanently deformed cells in the peripheral blood, so that the absolute numbers of these cells is not a determinant of clinical status. It may be, however, that their turnover rate, about which little is known, is a determining factor. Much information remains to be gathered as to why some patients do so well and some do so poorly; and it is apparent that this information probably will not come out of routine morphologic observations of the peripheral blood.

Any comments on the pathogenesis of the sickle syndromes must necessarily include considerations of hemoglobins other than Hb S present in red cells. For example, it is well known that a certain amount of fetal hemoglobin (Hb F) present in red cells along with Hb S prolongs the life of that red cell and presumably provides some sort of favorable influence on the clinical state of the host. Although no clear-cut relationship between Hb F levels and clinical course exists in most Hb SS individuals, there is increasing evidence that levels as high as 15%, despite the fact that Hb F may not be homogeneously distributed from cell to cell, may be remarkably beneficial (Perrine et al., 1972). This variability in amounts of Hb F from cell to cell in any one population of Hb SS erythrocytes is rather clearly demonstrated in Figure 5. This is known as a "Betke preparation" wherein hemoglobins other than Hb F are eluted from slide preparations of peripheral blood; and, hence after staining of the remaining cells, the amount of fetal hemoglobin is revealed by the density of the stain in individual cells. This is a semiquantitative estimation of the amount of Hb F at best, but demonstrates the wide variability in Hb F from cell to cell. Note that the permanently deformed cells are, by and large, low in Hb F. Corroboration of this finding can be achieved by centrifuging out, at high speed, these permanently deformed cells. Direct analysis of the amount of Hb F contained in them demonstrate that, whereas total hemoglobin per cell appears to be constant, the amount of Hb F in the permanently deformed cells is low.

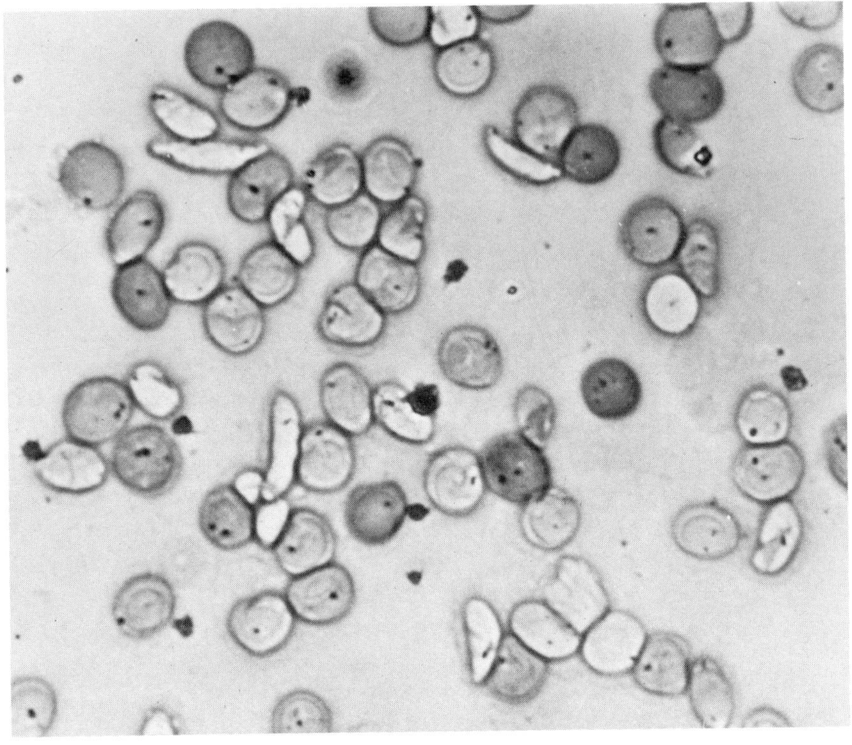

Fig. 5. Photomicrograph of oxygenated Hb SS erythrocytes stained for Hb F by the "Betke technique." A variability of Hb F from cell to cell is noted, and the permanently deformed cells (ISC) are low in Hb F. From Bertles and Milner, 1968.

The most reasonable explanation of this finding is that low proportions of Hb F in an erythrocyte facilitate sickle-unsickle cycles, hence leading to permanent deformation by mechanisms described above. Certain individuals working on hemoglobinopathies feel that there may be a possibility of capitalizing on this variability in the amount of Hb F synthesized from cell to cell. If, somehow, it were possible to raise the amount of Hb F to, say, 15% in *each* cell in the circulation of an Hb SS individual, red cell life span would probably be close to normal and the patient would be asymptomatic or nearly so. Experience with patients who are doubly heterozygous for Hb S and for hereditary persistence of fetal hemoglobin (HPFH) supports this contention, for in these individuals the increased amounts of Hb F *are* homogeneously distributed from cell to cell, and the individuals themselves, although bearing high proportions of Hb S, are asymptomatic. There is still a wealth of information yet to be gleaned about the distribution and interaction of various hemoglobins within Hb SS cells, concentrations of hemoglobins in SS cells, characteristics and composition of red cell membrane, and the behavior of Hb SS erythrocytes in the microcirculation.

Further emphasis on Hb F as a pathogenetically important instrument in other hemoglobinopathies is provided by the graphic comparison of homozygous β-thalassemia with Hb SS disease in Figure 6. Patients' blood, in both situations, has been centrifuged to give dense cells and light cells. In thalassemia, hemoglobin per cell is uniformly low, and those cells carrying the high proportion of Hb F (the dense cells which go to the bottom of the centrifuge) have the longest life span. In Hb SS disease, the denser (older) cells contain the greater amounts of Hb F, but the densest cells (bar to the far right) are predominantly ISC; and these relatively short-lived cells contain lesser amounts of Hb F. The *basic* difference between β thalassemia and Hb SS disease is, of course, the fact that in thalassemia there is decreased synthesis of β-chains, whereas in Hb SS disease there is synthesis of relatively normal amounts of an abnormal β chain. The important similarity between the two diseases is the fact that the presence of Hb F within erythrocytes provides an ameliorating influence. This important point has not been lost on a number of research teams, and considerable attention is now being paid in several laboratories to the possibility of augmenting synthesis of Hb F. In terms of biochemical genetics, this implies derepressing synthesis of γ chains.

Any discussion of pathogenesis in the sickle cell syndromes necessarily includes an examination of precisely what is going on inside the abnormal erythrocytes.

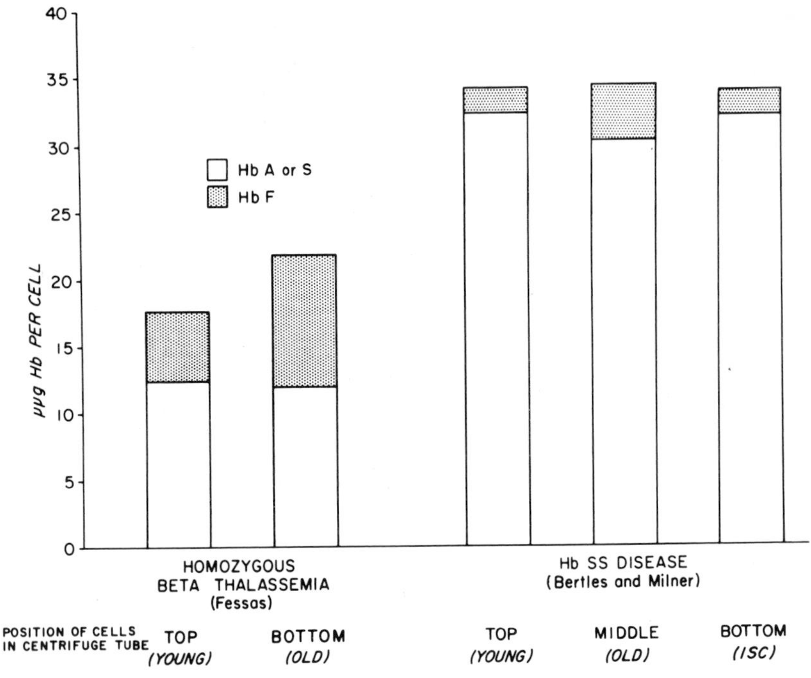

Fig. 6. Comparison of homozygous β-thalassemia and Hb SS disease. In both diseases, cells relatively rich in Hb F are selected for survival (right bar in β-thalassemia; middle bar in Hb SS disease). Whereas hemoglobin per cell is low in β-thalassemia, it is normal in Hb SS erythrocytes regardless of cell size, shape, or ultracentrifugal behavior. See text for details. From Bertles, 1973.

Figure 7 is a thin-section electron micrograph of an oxygenated Hb SS erythrocyte which, indeed, looks completely normal. There are no intracellular inclusions, and the general shape of the cell is normal.

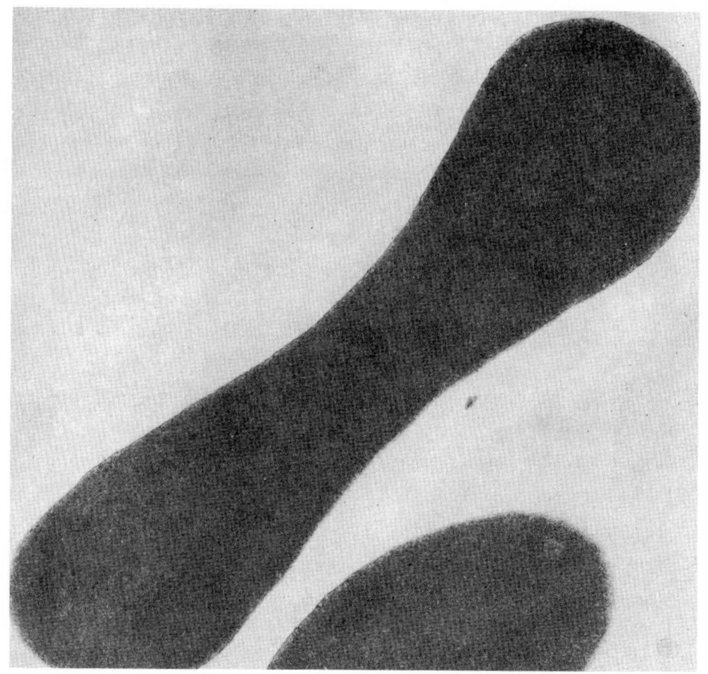

Fig. 7. Thin-section electron micrograph of an oxygenated non-deformed Hb SS erythrocyte. From Bertles and Döbler, 1969.

As deoxygenation proceeds (Fig. 8), fibers composed of deoxygenated molecules of Hb S are formed, lying parallel within the protuberances of the cell. When deoxygenation is nearly complete (Fig. 9), a regularity of fiber bundle formation is apparent, the bundles extending approximately in the long axis of the deoxygenated Hb SS cell. Although forces known to be responsible for the aggregation of deoxygenated molecules of Hb S are so-called "weak" forces, bundles of these fibers are apparently strong enough to warp deoxygenated cells into the well-known sickle silhouette. Whether in cells or in cell-free solution, the fibers have the same transverse dimension (170 Å). In bundles, they have the same center-to-center distance (approximately 225 Å).

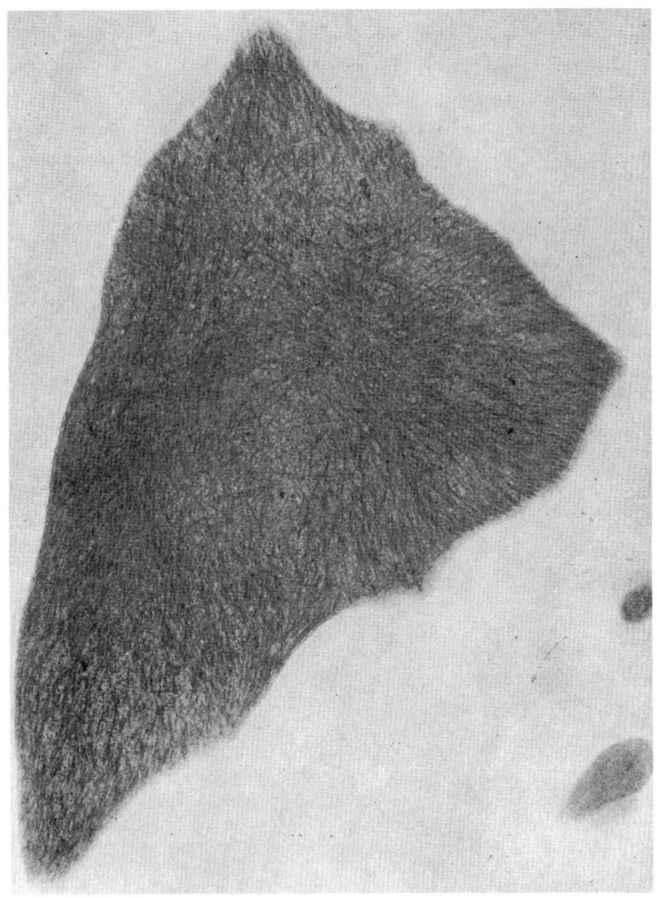

Fig. 8. Thin-section electron micrograph of a partiall deoxygenated Hb SS erythrocyte. From Bertles and Döble 1969.

Most recently (Finch et al., 1973), what may be a fairly accurate representation has been educed of how individual deoxygenated molecules of Hb S aggregate to form these fibers (Fig. 10). The globes in the figure are deoxygenated molecules of Hb S. Each fiber appears to be a tube made up of six thin filaments wound around the tubular surface with a pitch of approximately 3,000 Å. The thin filaments are strings of single hemoglobin molecules.

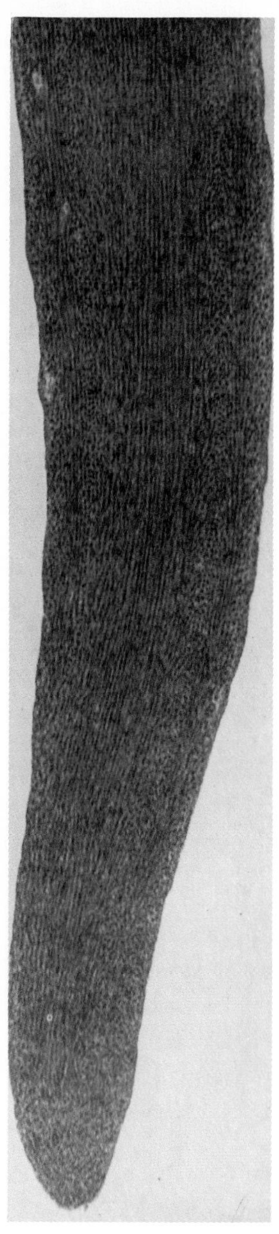

Fig. 9. Thin-section electron micrograph of a more completely deoxygenated Hb SS erythrocyte. From Bertles and Döbler, 1969.

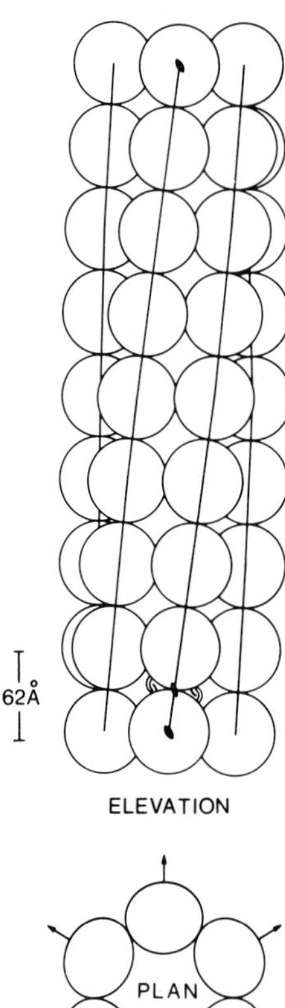

Fig. 10. Three-dimensional structure of a fiber composed of deoxygenated molecules (the spheres in the drawing) of Hb S. The fiber may be viewed as six helical strings of Hb S molecules, or alternatively as a stack of six-membered disks. Fibers aggregate in bundles to form the structures seen in Figures 8 and 9. From Finch et al., 1973.

Alternatively, the fiber may be thought of as a stack of six-membered disks, each disk rotated slightly upon the next to generate six helices. Note that, in this model, each molecule contacts four of its neighbors. Searches are now under way in a number of laboratories to determine precisely these contact regions.

Thus these two small mutational changes in each Hb S molecule that you have heard about elsewhere in this symposium, comprised of a substitution of valine for glutamate at one point in each of the two β chains, is responsible, ultimately, for the syndrome of sickle cell disease in all its complexity. Molecules of Hb S, when deoxygenated, aggregate into fibers; the fibers arrange themselves in bundles; the bundles warp the cell into a semi-rigid facsimile of a sickle or scythe; other Hb SS cells, even when not deoxygenated, develop abnormal membranes and a dangerously increased internal viscosity; passage through the microcirculation is impeded; tissues are deprived of their oxygen supply; and the end result is a very sick human being deserving of all the care, attention, and research efforts that we can bring to bear on this problem.

QUESTIONS AND ANSWERS

1. *Is there any evidence that platelet function or life span is abnormal in sickle cell disease?*
   It has been obvious for some years that patients with Hb SS disease have an increase in their platelet count. However, only recently has there been a study on platelet survival in these patients (Haut et al., 1973). Haut and his co-workers found that platelet survival in Hb SS patients who are not in crisis and are without obvious complications is normal. Platelet aggregation is also normal in these patients. However, platelet survival in patients in crisis was significantly shortened. This increased thrombopoiesis during crisis persists after the crisis has subsided and causes, for a short time, an even higher platelet count than before. Haut and his co-workers felt that it was too early to say whether or not platelets play an active role in the pathogenesis of some of the sickle syndromes.

2. *Do you think that capillary walls themselves are involved in the pathogenesis of sickle disease?*

Diggs (1973) makes the strong point that stasis in small blood vessels favors hypoxia and this leads on to endothelial proliferation. Hence, the lumina of terminal blood vessels are narrowed, contributing to the vasoocculusive process.

3. *When Hb SS cells are repetitively deoxygenated and oxygenated, do the fibers form in exactly the same place?* The experimental design to answer your question simply does not yet exist. The electron micrographs I have shown here in this portion of the symposium all have been thin sections of fixed cells. Hence, one cannot tell yet whether local effects within the cell may induce fiber formation in exactly the same way from time to time.

4. *We have already heard earlier from Dr. Nagel some information about possible contact areas between deoxygenated molecules of Hb S. I wonder if your ideas correspond with his?* Certainly there are some constraints to intermolecular contact that cannot be neglected: for example, the β6 regions. It appears also that β121 and β73 must somehow be involved, either at contact regions or somehow influencing them. Dr. Nagel and his colleagues have done excellent work with Hb C Harlem, work which has led us into interesting concepts of how these molecules may fit together. An attack on this problem going on in our own laboratories might be described briefly here. My colleague, Dr. Magdoff-Fairchild, is supplying a computer with the position of each atom in a deoxygenated molecule of hemoglobin and then asking the computer to calculate, in effect, X-ray diffraction patterns of a series of hypothetical fibers in which the orientation of the hemoglobin molecule is systematically varied. As this search procedure goes on, the computer-generated patterns are compared to actual X-ray diffraction patterns. Eventually, with the help of this and information gathered from other sources we hope to identify the contact regions between Hb S molecules. The clinical goal, of course, is to

find some way of interrupting the fit between these Hb S molecules so that fibers cannot form. It must be admitted that neither the computer work nor the concept of finding a way of stopping intermolecular fit are simple ones.

5. *I have a question about the so-called "Finch model" (Fig. 10). The arrows in the disk (Fig. 10) imply that the molecular dyad, i.e., the Y-axis of each molecule in the disk is arranged radially to the center of the fiber. I wonder what the basis for this arrangement is?* At the time the model you speak of was drawn, it seemed reasonable and simpler to draw the molecules with the Y-axes in that direction. However, further information makes it unlikely, and we are looking at other orientations.

6. (Question by Dr. Rucknagel): *I agree with your general picture of the microcirculation that you presented. And that is where I have been through in my own thinking; but, something bothers me about it. That is, on microscopic examination, or, say autopsy data, we don't see a lot of evidence for general microcirculation impairment. We see some problems in the lung, and some of these are pulmonary emboli. We, of course, have the problem of the spleen, but we almost never see skin thrombosis. I've looked at a lot of muscle sections and haven't seen microcirculation impairment there. We do see it in the bone, of course.* I think Dr. Rucknagel is right. There is much more to be learned about both the micro= and macrocirculation in the sickle syndromes. Although it does appear reasonable to think of this as a "small vessel disease," autopsy material simply does not always bear this out, although certainly Dr. Diggs has quite a bit of evidence in the direction of this being chiefly small vessel. The truth of the matter is that very frequently pathological examination does not explain clinical situations.

7. *Since you say that fetal hemoglobin is advantageous in this disease, does it help to transfuse red cells high in fetal hemoglobin to these patients?* If transfusion becomes mandatory, the best course is to give normal (AA) red cells. They're made for adults, and they work very well. There is no point in giving cells high in fetal hemoglobin, for they would not function any better than AA red cells and conceptually might even function less effectively. My point about fetal hemoglobin was that it should be inside the cells carrying Hb S, for fetal hemoglobin appears to reduce fiber formation and, consequently, sickling, when present at high enough concentrations in Hb SS red cells.

REFERENCES

1. Bertles, J.F., 1973. *Multiple Hemoglobins in Cells: Significance and Genetic Control.* In Sickle Cell Disease; Abramson, Bertles, and Wethers, eds. C.V. Mosby, St. Louis, 1973, 71.

2. Bertles, J.F., and Döbler, J., 1969. *Reversible and Irreversible Sickling: A Distinction by Electron Microscopy.* Blood 33:884.

3. Bertles, J.F., and Milner, P.F.A., 1968. *Irreversibly Sickled Erythrocytes: A Consequence of the Heterogeneous Distribution of Hemoglobin Types in Sickle-cell Anemia.* J. Clin. Invest. 47:1731.

4. Burton, A.C., 1966. *Role of Geometry, of Size and Shape, in the Microcirculation.* Federation Proceedings 25:1753.

5. Cameron, A.A.C., McCord, C.W., and Bertles, J.F., 1971. *Successful Replacement of Aortic and Mitral Valves with Ball Valve Prostheses in a Patient with Rheumatic Heart Disease and SC Hemoglobinopathy.* Am. J. Cardiology 27:318.

6. Chien, S., Usami, S., and Bertles, J.F., 1970. *Abnormal Rheology of Oxygenated Blood in Sickle Cell Anemia.* J. Clin. Invest. 49:623.

7. Diggs, L.W., 1973. *Anatomic Lesions in Sickle Cell Disease.* In Sickle Cell Disease: Abramson, Bertles, and Wethers, eds., C.V. Mosby, St. Louis, 1973, 189.

8. Eaton, J.W., Skelton, T.D., Swofford, H.S., Kolpin, C.E., and Jacob, H.S., 1973. *Elevated Erythrocyte Calcium in Sickle Cell Disease.* Nature 246:105.

9. Finch, J.T., Perutz, M.F., Bertles, J.F., and Döbler, J., 1973. *Structure of Sickle-cell Hemoglobin Fibers.* Proc. Nat. Acad. Sci. USA 70:718.

10. Haut, M.J., Cowan, D.H., and Harris, J.W., 1973. *Platelet Function and Survival in Sickle Cell Disease.* J. Lab. Clin. Med. 82:44.

11. Jensen, M., Shohet, S.B., and Nathan, D.G., 1973. *The Role of Red Cell Energy Metabolism in the Generation of Irreversibly Sickled Cells in vitro.* Blood 42:835.

12. Jensen, W.N., and Klug, P.P., 1973. *Cell Membrane in Sickle Cell Disease.* In Sickle Cell Disease: Abramson, Bertles, and Wethers, eds. C.V. Mosby, St. Louis, 1973, 130.

13. Perrine, R.P., Brown, M.J., Weatherall, D.J., Clegg, J.B., and May, A., 1972. *Benign Sickle-cell Anemia.* The Lancet 1163.

14. Seakins, M., Gibbs, W.N., Milner, P.F., and Bertles, J.F., 1973. *Erythrocyte Hb S Concentration: An Important Factor in the Low Oxygen Affinity of Blood in Sickle Cell Anemia.* J. Clin. Invest. 52:422.

CLINICAL ASPECTS
OF
SICKLE CELL DISEASE

Margaret G. Robinson, M.D.

The clinical aspects of sickle hemoglobinopathy in adults is becoming common knowledge. The major medical problems and the natural history of the disease during childhood is less well known. Such knowledge is essential if the mortality and morbidity is to be decreased. For this reason, we have reviewed the records of the 693 children with various forms of Sickle Cell Disease (exclusive of Sickle Cell Trait) who were seen by the pediatric hematology section of Kings County Hospital/Downstate Medical Centers. Because of possible bias being introduced by including patients who were rendered only emergency care, only those children who had died or who had been followed in the pediatric hematology and the comprehensive pediatric sickle cell clinics for 6 months or more were included in this review (Table 1).

TABLE 1. *SICKLE HEMOGLOBINOPATHY PATIENTS SEEN IN PEDIATRICS AT KINGS COUNTY HOSPITAL, JANUARY, 1956 - DECEMBER, 1973.*

Hemoglobin Type	Total No. Of Patients	Patients Followed More Than 6 Months*	Patient Years	Average Years Of Follow-up
SS	513	420	1882	4.5
SC	99	74	228	3.0
S-β-Thalassemia	78	57	194	3.4
S-HPFH	1			
S-D**	1			
S-α-Thalassemia	1			
TOTAL:	693	551	2304	4.2

*Includes 11 patients who died less than 6 months following diagnosis.
**Probably represents Hb SD; work-up not completed.

Of these remaining 551 patients, 420 (76.3%) were Hb SS, 74 (13.4%) were Hb SC, and 57 (10.3%) were Hb-S-β-thalassemia by electrophoretic studies. The 383 living Hb SS patients were followed from 6 months to 16 years with an average of 4.8 years. The remaining 37 Hb SS patients who had died were followed from 1 day to 15 years with a mean follow-up of 1.8 years. The total number of years of follow-up for these children was 1886 patient-years. The 74 Hb SC children were followed for 6 months to 11½ years (mean of 3 years) for a total of 228 patient-years while the 57 Hb S-thalassemia children were followed for an average of 3.4 years (6 months to 12 years) and a total of 193.5 patient-years.

MORTALITY DATA

To determine the major problems, the mortality data was examined (Tables 2 and 3).

TABLE 2. *DEATHS IN SICKLE HEMOGLOBINOPATHY*

A. PERCENT MORTALITY BY HEMOGLOBIN TYPE:

Hemoglobin Type	No. of Deaths	% Mortality
SS	37	8.8
SC	0	0.0
S-Thalassemia	3	5.3
TOTAL:	40	7.3

B. PERCENT OF TOTAL DEATHS BY AGE:

Age (Years)	No.	% Of Total Deaths
Under 1	9	22.5
1-3	18	45
4-8	8	20.0
9-13	3	7.5
14-22	2	5.0
Under 4 Years	27	67.5
Over 4 Years	17	32.5

TABLE 3.

CAUSES OF DEATH IN SICKLE HEMOGLOBINOPATHY

			No.	%
1.	*INFECTIONS:*		26*	65
	Sepsis	11		
	Pneumonia	7		
	Meningitis	4		
	Diarrhea	2		
	Myocarditis	2		
2.	*CENTRAL NERVOUS SYSTEM PROBLEMS:*		17*	42.5
	Meningitis	4		
	CVA-thrombotic	10		
	CVA-hemorrhagic	3		
3.	*SEQUESTRATION:*		7*	17.5
4.	*DOA*		2	5.0
5.	*DISSEMINATED COAGULOPATHY*		2	5.0
6.	*CONGENITAL HEART DISEASE*		2	5.0
7.	*APLASTIC CRISIS*		1	2.5
8.	*POST-SPLENECTOMY INFECTION SYNDROME*		1	2.5
9.	*RENAL FAILURE*		1	2.5
10.	*TRAUMA*		1	2.5

*Primary Cause - Infections - 19, CNS-11, Sequestration-6, DIC-2, Renal Failure-1, Trauma-1.

Forty children (37 Hb SS and 3 Hb S-thalassemia) died for an overall mortality of 7.3% and for only the Hb SS children, 8.8%. There was no significant sex differential (22 females, 18 males). A striking age difference was seen, the majority (67.5%) of the deaths occurring under 4 years and 87.5% under the age of 9 years. The major causes of death either as the primary or as an associated cause were infections (65%), central nervous system problems (42.5%), and sequestration crises (17.5%).

INFECTIONS

Not only were infections the principal cause of death, but they were second only to thrombotic crises as the reason for hospitalization. Almost 2/3 of the Hb SS, ½ of the Hb SC and 2/5 of the Hb S-thalassemia children had one or more of the infections listed in Table 4.

TABLE 4. *INCIDENCE AND TYPES OF INFECTIONS IN SICKLE HEMOGLOBINOPATHY*

	No. (%) Of Patients By Hemoglobin Type			
Infections	Hb SS	Hb S-Thal.	Hb SC	Total
1. *PNEUMONIAS*	207 (49.3)	15 (26.3)	29 (39.2)	251 (45.5)
More than 1 episode	114	9	8	131
2. *DIARRHEA*	70 (16.7)	9 (15.8)	12 (16.2)	91 (16.5)
More than 1 episode	21	1	1	23
3. *URINARY TRACT INFECTIONS*	45 (10.7)	4 (7.0)	3 (4.0)	52 (9.4)
More than 1 episode	9	0	0	9
4. *MENINGITIS*	35 (8.3)	0	3 (4.0)	38 (6.9)
More than 1 episode	5	0	0	5
5. *SEPSIS*	22 (5.2)	2 (3.5)	2 (2.7)	26 (4.7)
6. *OSTEOMYELITIS*	14 (3.3)	0	0	14 (2.5)
7. *INFECTIOUS MONONUCLEOSIS*	13 (3.1)	1 (1.8)	2 (2.7)	16 (2.9)
8. *TUBERCULOSIS*	12 (2.9)	0	0	12 (2.2)
9. *TYPHOID FEVER*	2 (0.5)	0	0	2 (0.4)
No. (%) of patients with one or more infections:	269 (64.0)	24 (42.1)	40 (54.0)	333 (60.4)

In contrast to tuberculosis, which had an incidence in sickle hemoglobinopathies similar to that seen in our non-sickle Black children, there was a marked increase of pneumonias, diarrheas, urinary tract infections (UTI), meningitis, sepsis, and osteomyelitis. The risk of repeated infections of the same type was high (1 in 2 for pneumonias, 1 in 4 for diarrhea, 1 in 6 for UTI, and 1 in 8 for meningitis).

Pneumonias. The etiologic agent associated with the majority of the pneumonias was not determined definitely since lung biopsies were not performed. The majority of the nose and throat cultures that revealed pathogens grew out pneumococcus. Some blood cultures were positive for E. Coli, Salmonella and Klebsiella species, while other etiologic agents were obtained from pleural fluid or by rising antibody titers. A few etiologic agents were inferred from finding Salmonella in stool cultures and E. Coli in urine cultures at the time of the pneumonia. Interestingly, of the Hb SS children, 7 had pneumonia with measles and 2 had pneumonia with chickenpox (Table 5).

TABLE 5.

ETIOLOGIC AGENTS OF PNEUMONIAS

Organism	No.
Pneumococcus	14
Gram Positive Organisms In Pleural Fluid Or Sputum	8
Measles	7
Escherichia Coli	7
Staphylococcus Aureus	6
Mycoplasma	5
Salmonella	4
Klebsiella-Enterobacter sp.	3
Hemophilus Influenzae	2
Chickenpox	2
Group Aβ-hemolytic Streptococcus	1

Repeated episodes of pneumonia were common. Eighty-one patients had 2 or 3 pneumonias, 21 children had 4 or 5 episodes, and 12 children had 6 to 18 attacks. Two of the children had 9 pneumonias in a 3 year period while one individual had 18 pneumonias in 15 years. None of these children showed any evidence of congenital anomalies of the lung, nor any hypogammaglobulinemia to explain these findings.

Although in the majority of children, the pneumonias responded clinically to adequate penicillin or ampicillin therapy in 5 to 7 days, roentgenographic changes of consolidation persisted for 2 to 4 weeks. This suggested that infarction may occur concurrently in the area of the pneumonia or may be the sole cause of the consolidation. One child following trauma to the chest was admitted to the hospital with a left lower lobe consolidation. Clinically, she had no evidence of infection. A radioisotope lung scan and blood flow studies revealed decreased uptake not only in the left lower lobe but also in the right lower lobe and the superior segment of the right upper lobe. These latter two filling defects were suggestive of old pulmonary infarcts.

As has been reported previously, Mycoplasma pneumonia in sickle cell disease produces an extensive consolidation and a protracted complicated clinical course unless treated promptly with erythromycin[1]. When these children do not respond clinically to the usual antibiotic therapy, Mycoplasma pneumonias and the gram negative organisms (E. Coli, H. Influenzae, Salmonella, Enterobacter-Klebsiella species, etc.) should be suspected of being the etiologic agent. Because of the high incidence of bacteremia, the organism producing a concurrent UTI or if the stool culture is positive for Salmonella, the pneumonia should be treated as if these were the causative agent.

Meningitis. Meningitis was diagnosed 45 times in 38 patients (Table 6) with two patients having 3 episodes and 3 patients having 2 episodes of pneumococcal meningits.

The incidence of meningits in Hb SS was 8.3% while that in Hb SC disease was 4.0%. No patient with Hb S-thalassemia had meningitis. The majority of the meningitides occurred prior to 4 years of age, an age when Hemophilus influenzae is the etiologic agent in almost half of the non-sickle children with meningitis seen at Kings County Hospital. In contrast, the pneumococcus was isolated from the cerebrospinal fluid in 56% of all the meningitides and in 83% of the proven bacterial meningitides. The marked increased incidence of meningitis, the finding of repeated episodes by different types of the pneumococcus, and the high incidence of the pneumococcus as the etiologic agent is similar to our previous published report and to that of Barrett-Connor's series of 166 Hb SS patients of all ages.[2,3]

An increased incidence of 2.41% of H. influenzae meningitis and sepsis was reported by Barrett-Connor.[3] In the Kings County series, there were only 2 patients with H. influenzae meningitis or sepsis and 2 with H. influenzae pneumoniae for an overall incidence of 0.95%.

Urinary Tract Infections. Urinary tract infections were encountered in 10.7% of Hb SS children, 7% of Hb S-thalassemia and 4% of Hb SC patients (Table 4) in contrast to the usual 2% during infancy and 1% in school age girls.[4] Multiple episodes were encountered in 1/5 of the Hb SS children. Intravenous pyelograms and voiding cystourethrograms revealed only 2 of the 52 children with urinary tract anomalies. The usual etiologic agent (approximately 90%) in UTI of a non-obstructive type in Hb AA children is E. Coli. Although E. Coli was found in nearly 47% of UTI in sickle hemoglobinopathy, 16% were caused by Enterobacter-Klebsiella species, almost 10% by Proteus, and 10% by multiple or unusual organism (Table 7). In her Florida series, Barrett-Connor encountered paracolon and Enterobacter-Klebsiella species as etiologic agent in 6 of 10 Hb SS and 1 Hb SC patient with UTI.[3,5]

TABLE 6.

ETIOLOGIC AGENTS OF MENINGITIS AND OSTEOMYELITIS

A. MENINGITIS:

Organism	No.
Pneumococcus	25
H. Influenzae	2
E. Coli	1
Staphylococcus Aureus	1
Streptococcus	1
Aseptic (Mumps, ECHO, etc.)	4
Partially Treated	11

B. OSTEOMYELITIS

Organism	No.
Salmonella	9
Staphylococcus Aureus	2
Pneumococcus	1
Unknown	4

TABLE 7

ETIOLOGIC AGENTS OF URINARY TRACT INFECTIONS

Organism	No.	%
Escherichia Coli	30	41.1
E. Coli & Proteus Species	3	4.1
E. Coli, Proteus and Pseudomonas	1	1.4
Klebsiella-Enterobacter	10	13.7
Klebsiella-Enterobacter and Proteus	2	2.7
Proteus sp.	1	1.4
Staphylococcus Aureus	1	1.4
Herella Vagincola	1	1.4
Unknown (Clinical Symptoms Plus Pyuria)	24	32.9
TOTAL:	73	100.1
All E. Coli	34	46.6
All Klebsiella-Enterobacter	12	16.4
All Proteus	7	9.6

Not only is there an overall increased incidence of UTI and an increased incidence of multiple or unusual etiologic agents without evidence of obstructive phenomenon, but it is also more difficult to eradicate the infection. Because of the high incidence of positive urine cultures for the same organism one week after a 2-week course of antibiotic therapy, for the past 10 years we have been treating all sickle children with UTI for a minimum of 6 weeks.

Osteomyelitis. The common finding of Salmonella osteomyelitis in sickle disease is familiar to physicians. Our incidence of osteomyelitis was 2.5% overall and 3.3% in Hb SS children. Two of the 14 patients had episodes of Salmonella osteomyelitis separated by 2 and 7 years. The etiologic agent was detected by blood cultures or by aspiration of pus from the point of maximal tenderness in 12 of the 16 episodes (Table 6). Nine were caused by Salmonella species, 2 by Staphylococcus aureus, and 1 by Streptococcus pneumoniae (Diplococcus pneumoniae). In the literature, other gram-negative organisms (E. Coli, Shigella, etc.) have been reported.[6,9] Barrett-Connor reported an incidence of 12.6% for osteomyelitis among her 166 Hb SS children and adults.[3] The reason for the marked difference in frequency between the Florida and Brooklyn series is unknown.

Clinically these patients are more toxic and have point tenderness over the involved area in contrast to the more diffuse pain of a thrombotic crisis. As a general rule, it is not possible to differentiate a crisis from osteomyelitis by x-ray. Both do not show bone changes until 10-17 days after onset and the changes seen are similar. Frequently, more than one bone is involved in contrast to osteomyelitis in Hb AA patients. In some cases of Salmonella sepsis or bacteremia, evidence of osteomyelitis are not seen for several weeks to months after the acute episode: *S.C. was a 13 year old, toxic-appearing child with diarrhea and a temperature of 105°F. Blood and stool cultures were positive for Salmonella typhimurium. Although she complained of back pain, no swelling or tenderness was found. Lumbothoracic x-rays taken 2 and 4 weeks after onset were negative for bone pathology. Three months later a repeat spine x-ray was obtained for evaluation of continued back pain. A collapsed vertebrae was found.*

Etiologic Agents. The organisms most frequently encountered were the pneumococcus, E. Coli, Salmonella, Enterobacter-Klebsiella, and Staphylococcus aureus (Table 8).

TABLE 8. *INCIDENCE AND ATTACK RATE OF ORGANISMS CAUSING SERIOUS INFECTIONS IN SICKLE HEMOGLOBINOPATHY*

	No.	%	Attack Rate Per 1000 Patient-years
A. Hb SS PATIENTS:			
Pneumococcus	38	9.0	20.19
E. Coli	33	7.9	17.53
Salmonella (Excluding Typhoid)	16	3.8	8.50
Enterobacter-Klebsiella Species	10	2.4	5.31
Staphylococcus Aureus	10	2.4	5.31
Group Aβ-hemolytic Streptococcus	9	2.1	4.78
Proteus Species	5	1.2	2.66
Mycoplasma	4	0.95	2.13
Hemophilus Influenzae	4	0.95	2.13
Pseudomonas Aeruginosa	2	0.48	1.06
Salmonella Typhosa	2	0.48	1.06
Shigella	1	0.24	0.53
Herella Vagincola	1	0.24	0.53
Meningococcus	1	0.24	0.53
Group Gβ-streptococcus	1	0.24	0.53
Bacteroides	1	0.24	0.53
Infectious Mononucleosis	13	3.1	6.91
Tuberculosis	12	2.9	6.38

B. Hb SC AND S-THALASSEMIA:	SC	S-THAL	TOTAL	Attack Rate Per 1000 Patient-years
Pneumococcus	2 (2.7%)	0	2	4.74
E. Coli	3 (4.1%)	1 (1.8%)	4	9.48
Enterobacter-Klebsiella	0	2 (3.5%)	2	4.74
Stap. Aureus	0	1 (1.8%)	1	2.37
Mycoplasma	0	1 (1.8%)	1	2.37
Paracolon	1 (1.4%)	0	1	2.37

The attack rate per 1,000 patient-years for the pneumococcus, Salmonella, and tuberculosis (20.19, 8.50, and 6.38 respectively) were similar to those found by Barrett-Connor in her series of Hb SS patients (namely 23.15, 8.10, and 5.79 respectively). However, the attack rate for H. influenzae was ½ and that for Shigella was 1/13 the rate found in the Florida series.[3]

Although enteropathogenic E. Coli diarrhea and E. Coli UTI accounted for 85% of the E. Coli infections, there were also several other unusual E. Coli infections (Tables 9 and 10).

TABLE 9

ESCHERICHIA COLI INFECTIONS IN SICKLE HEMOGLOBINOPATHY

TOTAL NUMBER OF INFECTIONS:	54*
U.T.I.	31
Enteropathogenic E. Coli Diarrhea	12
Pneumonias	7
Infection of Surgical and Traumatic Wounds	4
Sepsis	3
Meningitis	1

*7 Infections Involved 2 Categories.

UNUSUAL E. COLI INFECTIONS FOR AGE AND/OR SITE

AGE	*SEX*	*DIAGNOSIS*	*COMMENTS*
6 Mos.	F	E. Coli Pneumonia & UTI	Had 9 pneumonias (1 H. Flu., 1 Staph. Aureus, 1 E. Coli, 6 no Organism Cultured; 4 UTI (All E. Coli), IVP-normal; 3 episodes of diarrhea; 1 Pneumococcal Meningitis; and 5 hand-foot crises in 3½ years. Died: Viral Myocarditis.
11 Mos.	F	E. Coli & Enterobacter Aerogenes Pneumoempyema Plus RLL Pneumonia	Died.
18 Mos.	M	E. Coli RML Pneumonia And UTI	Had LLL Pneumonia-Age 11 mos., RLL Pneumonia; Age-23 mos.
4¼ Yrs.	F	E. Coli RML Pneumonia And UTI	Hemolytic crisis associated with it (Hb 4.2, Retic 19.9%, spleen not palpable, WBC 49,500) plus one other pneumonia in 4¼ years.
5 Yrs.	M	E. Coli Meningitis And Sepsis	CSF and blood cultures positive. T-105°F. Aplastic crisis-Hb 5.0, Retic 0.1%, B.M.-decreased erythroid precursors. Also had 1 episode of diarrhea, 10 pneumonias (2 with purulent pleural effusions) in 8 years.
7½ Yrs.	F	E. Coli Bilateral Lower Lobe Pneumonia Plus Pleural Effusion On Right	T-104°F, septic course. Also had Salmonellosis-septic type, plus another pneumonia in 8 years.

TABLE 10.
(Continued)

AGE	*SEX*	*DIAGNOSIS*	*COMMENTS*
10 Yrs.	M	Enteropathogenic E. Coli	T-104°F, culture negative for S & S; also had 1 pneumonia; 2 E. Coli UTI, 1 Klebsiella UTI (IVP normal); subacute endocarditis and pericardial effusion. Died.
12½ Yrs.	M	E. Coli Cellulitis Of Foot (traumatic puncture by nail)	Also had meningitis, age 8.
15 Yrs.	F	E. Coli Pneumonia & UTI	Hb 3.5gm%, WBC 2800, B.M.-increased early precursors with arrest at basophilic stage and maturation arrest of myeloid series. Aplastic crisis.
16 Yrs.	F	E. Coli UTI and Sepsis	T-105°F, septic course; blood and urine cultures positive; had 2 episodes of pneumonia previously.
17 Yrs.	M	Enteropathogenic E. Coli 0119:B14 Diarrhea	T-104°F, also aplastic crisis (Hb 5.5gm%, retic 3.7%, retic production index = 0.6); has had numerous painful crises, gallstones and nephrotic syndrome but no other serious infections.

There was a mixed E. Coli-enterobacter aerogenes pneumoempyema in an 11 month old infant, an E. Coli sepsis and meningitis in a 5 year old, and E. Coli pleural effusion and pneumonia in a 7½ year old, 2 enteropathogenic E. Coli diarrheas with septic courses in a 10 year old and a 17 year old, and an E. Coli post-traumatic cellulitis of the foot in a 12 year old. The finding of these E. Coli infections in unusual sites or ages is highly suggestive of a marked increased susceptibility of Hb SS patients to this organism. In recent prospective study of infection in sickle cell anemia, we have confirmed this restrospective impression.[10]

The problems of a high frequency of bacteremia in all forms of infections and of overwhelming sepsis with death occurring within 2-3 hours up to 3 days of onset of their symptoms necessitates intensive antibiotic therapy for all infections in these children. Because of the increased attack rate by gram-negative enterics and H. influenzae as well as the pneumococcus organism, a broad spectrum bacteriocidal antibiotic should be used at maximum dosage for the first 2-3 days. Our current preference is ampicillin in dosages of 150-200 mg/kg/day given intravenously in divided doses every 4 hours for the first 2 days before reducing the dosage. Once the etiologic agent has been identified, therapy can be adjusted according to the sensitivities obtained and the clinical state of the patient. Only by doing this can we hope to decrease the following occurrences: *A 2 year old Hb SS lad awoke at 7:00 a.m. with mild respiratory distress and a temperature of 101°F. He arrived in the emergency room at 9:00 a.m. where he was found to have a few rales in both lower bases posteriorly. He did not appear toxic. Following a visit to the x-ray department, he arrived on the ward at 10:30 a.m. His temperature was 102°F but there was no other change in his clinical state. His hemogram was in the range that he normally had. Penicillin, 500,000 units q 6 h i.m. was ordered and one dose was administered by 11:30 a.m. He ate lunch and at 1:30 p.m. he had a cardio-respiratory arrest and was in shock. Post-mortem examination revealed evidence of sepsis with very early evidence of meningitis. Blood cultures obtained antemortem were positive for H. influenzae.*

CRISES

Sickle hemoglobinopathy patients are subject to 3 types of crises: thrombotic, aplastic, and sequestration. In infancy and early childhood, the thrombotic crisis has a propensity to involve the dorsum of the hands and feet in a relatively symmetrical fashion. It is uncommon to have only 1 or 3 extremities involved. This type of crisis occurs in 31.9% of Hb SS, 14% of Hb S-thalassemia, and 9% of Hb SC children (Table 11).

TABLE 11. *INCIDENCE OF OTHER CLINICAL PROBLEMS*

	Hb SS		*Hb SC*		*Hb S-THALASSEMIA*		*TOTAL*
	No.	*%*	*No.*	*%*	*No.*	*%*	*%*
Hand-foot	134	31.9	7	9.5	8	14.0	27
Aseptic Necrosis Of Femur	8	1.9	1	1.4	0		1.6
Aseptic Necrosis Head Of Humerus	1	0.2	0		0		0.2
Ulcers	14	3.3	2	2.7	1	1.8	3.1
Gallstones	13	3.1	0		0		2.4
Priapism	7	3.4	1	2.9	0		3.0

In our previous publication, we had quoted a 10.9% incidence in Hb SS patients but the present series more closely approximates the incidence seen in Africa.[11,12] The onset and recurrences of these hand-foot crises is predominantly under 3 years of age, rarely after 4 years. In 5 of our patients, their last episode occurred at 8 to 13 years of age. The pain and fever last from 5 to 10 days; the non-pitting swelling, from 1 to 4 weeks. The temperature in the milder forms is generally under 103°F but in the more severe episodes may be 104-105°F.

CENTRAL NERVOUS SYSTEM PROBLEMS

Thrombotic crises may occur any place in the body. When they occur in the brain, meninges or the blood supply to the spinal cord, neurologic signs and symptoms occur. Central nervous system problems were the second major cause of death in our patients and are a major management problem regardless of age. Two relatively large series of sickle patients reported in the literature quote a 35 to 40% incidence of central nervous system involvement.[13,14] The overall incidence in our children was 36% with 38% in the Hb SS children, 28% in Hb S-thalassemia, and 27% in the Hb SC patients (Table 12). The frequency and types of problems encountered are listed in Table 13.

TABLE 12.

INCIDENCE OF CENTRAL NERVOUS SYSTEM PROBLEMS

	ALL PROBLEMS		*CVA's*	
	No.	*%*	*No.*	*%*
Hb SS	160	38.1	35	8.3
Hb SC	20	27.0	2	2.7
Hb S-Thalassemia	16	28.1	0	0.0
TOTAL:	196	35.6	37	6.7

TABLE 13.

TYPES OF CENTRAL NERVOUS SYSTEM PROBLEMS

PROBLEM		*No.*	*%*
Headaches		55	10.1
Meningitis		38	6.9
CVA		37	6.7
CVA (Due to Hemorrhage)		4	
Convulsions		32	5.8
Plumbism		31	5.6
Nuchal Rigidity		31	5.6
Hemiplegia		18	3.3
Vertigo ("Dizziness, " Syncope, Ataxia)		17	3.1
Speech Problems		13	2.4
Expressive Aphasia		4	
Motor or Mental Retardation		11	2.6
Qudriplepia		9	1.6
Facial Palsy		7	1.3
Bell's Palsy	1		
Deafness (Sensioneural)		7	1.3
Behavior Problems		7	1.3
Minimal Brain Dysfunction	2		
Visual Disturbance		7	1.3
Strabismus Sudden Onset	1		
Hyphema	1		
Blindness	6		
Drowsiness, Lethargy		5	0.9
Opisthotonus		3	0.5
Hypertension		3	0.5
Psychic Reactions		3	0.5
Catatonia	1		
Hallucinations (Tactile)	1		
Visual	1		
Monoplegia		2	0.4
Tinnitus		2	0.4

Transient sensory loss, paresthesias of hands, Reyes syndrome, Guillam-Barre syndrome Parotid and facial swelling associated with severe headache..............................1 Each.

Frequent severe headaches, poorly responsive to analgesics, not infrequently accompanied by other painful crises, nuchal rigidity, or even transient hypertension was the most common complaint in our series and in that of Patterson et al.[14] Following an epistaxis or lumbar puncture, the headaches would abate.

Convulsions occurred as a part of meningitis, cerebrovascular accidents (CVA's), lead encephalopathy and as isolated events with no obvious etiology or sequelae. The incidence of convulsions in our series was twice that seen in the adults followed by Patterson.[14] This probably reflects the higher incidence of meningitis and lead encephalopathy encountered in children.

Nuchal rigidity unassociated with meningitis, upper respiratory tract infections, cervical adenitis or pneumonia occurred in almost 5% of the children. Initially we attributed this to infarction of the cervical vertebrae. In the few patients studied, vertebral roentgenograms revealed no change in the bony architecture on admission or 10 to 14 days later.

The vertigo, dizzy spells and syncope were not accompanied by a decrease in the patient's usual hemoglobin level. In one patient, the EEG showed the typical 3 per second spike and dome pattern of petit mal. These dizzy spells probably reflect cerebellar and vestibular dysfunction or "petit mal" like attacks resulting from minor CNS thrombotic crises.

Unexplained transitory hypertension was encountered in 3 patients in association with nuchal rigidity or severe headaches. When the nuchal rigidity or headache abated, the blood pressure returned to normal in 2 of the 3 patients. The third patient died (see next page). Renal investigation revealed no cause for the hypertension.

Transitory opisthotonous accompanied unexplained nuchal rigidity in 3 children disappearing when the neck pain and stiffness ceased. The psychic reactions consisted of one child with catatonia lasting 3 days, and 2 children with sensory hallucinations without evidence of infection or intoxication. Psychiatric evaluation of these children was consistent with a chronically ill child. Paresthesias of the hand and a transitory loss of tactile sensation were seen in 2 patients. Girdle-like radiculopathies reported in adults [13] were not seen in our patients.

Fortunately, the frequency of severe cerebrovascular accidents is relatively low (6.9% overall with 8.3% in Hb SS and 2.7% in Hb SC children) and is similar to that seen by Greer and Schotland (Hb SS 9.6%; Hb SC 3.4%)[13]. Unfortunately, those patients who have one CVA tend to have multiple episodes. One third of the Hb SS children with CVA's had 2 to 5 CVA's. With each successive episode, the morbidity and the risk of mortality increased. The sequellae seen following the cerebrovascular accidents included monoplegia, hemiplegia, quadriplegia, facial palsies, blindness, deafness, speech problems, mental and motor retardation, and behavior problems: *R.R., at age 2¼ years was admitted to the hospital with a flaccid left arm and left leg, a nasal twang to his speech and a left facial paresis. Radioisotope brain scan with blood flow studies and cerebroangiography demonstrated obstruction of the right middle cerebral artery. Eight months later he became stuporous, then comatose with decerebrate rigidity. He developed generalized seizures and cardiac arrest. Angiography on this occasion demonstrated bilateral anterior cerebral artery thrombosis.*

C.D., had pneumococcal meningitis at 1 11/12 years, developed right sided hemiparesis and right facial palsy at 2 8/12 years. The angiogram showed a left middle cerebral artery thrombosis. Four months later she developed sudden onset of total blindness. The pupils did not react to light and were dilated. The fundoscopic examination was normal. One month later, she had a left sided convulsion, nuchal rigidity, opisthotonus, a blood pressure of 130/90, and a temperature of 104°F. All cultures, including the spinal fluid were negative. She developed microscopic hematuria followed by gastrointestinal bleeding. Coagulation studies were consistent with a disseminated intravascular coagulopathy. She became comatose and died. Postmortem examination was refused.

We strongly believe that whenever possible, the diagnosis of CVA's should be made by lumbar puncture, EEG, and radioisotope brain scans with blood flow studies rather than by angiographic techniques. The radio-opaque dye used in cerebral angiography is hyperosmolar. Angiographic studies performed without transfusing the patient to a hemoglobin of 10-12 Gm% increases the risk of precipitating another CVA or having the present thrombus propagate further. Transfusing the patient increases his risk of developing hepatitis which the Hb SS patient handles poorly. Usually the radioisotope studies give all the necessary information for the diagnosis.

LESS COMMON THROMBOTIC CRISES

Aseptic Necrosis. Aseptic necrosis of the head of the femur (Table 11) is a relatively uncommon problem in the pediatric sickle hemoglobinopathy patient but presents a major management problem. It occurs with equal frequency in males and females, is more common over 10 years of age, tends to involve the left femur more often than the right, but may be bilateral. Destruction of the femoral head is progressive unless the patient can be kept at rest without weight bearing for 6 months to 1 year. This is relatively easily done in young children. Adolescents, however, refuse to stay in bed and, while using crutches, put weight on the affected hip. The newer hip replacement operations offer hope for relief of the crippling arthritic complications these patients can develop.

Priapism. During childhood, priapism, another difficult management problem, occurs in a relatively low frequency (3% of male sickle hemoglobinopathy children). The frequency increases with age and the symptomatology tends to become more severe in intensity and duration. In the young child, priapism generally lasts from hours to days, while in the adolescent it lasts from days to weeks and may ultimately lead to decreased fertility. We found fluid replacement, blood transfusions, and low molecular weight dextran unsuccessful in stopping the crisis. When taken orally on a daily basis, sodium bicarbonate 100 mg/kg or enough to keep the urine pH between 7.0 and 8.0 decreased the frequency of attacks in 2 patients but had no effect on the crises per se. Cyanate therapy tried in our oldest patient with priapism was beneficial. However, cyanate therapy is experimental, and although beneficial in one patient, there is not enough evidence that it will be of therapeutic value.

Ulcers. Typical stasis ulcers around the maleolus occurred in some of our children. In addition, ulcers which healed poorly occurred following an intramuscular injection in the buttock and following intravenous hydrating solution infiltrating into the wrist. Transfusions to obtain hemoglobin levels of 9-11 gm% and bed rest were used in the past for healing these ulcers. Currently, the direct administration of oxygen by mask to the ulcer has proved beneficial without transfusions.

Hematuria. Thrombotic episodes in the kidney ultimately lead to renal complications, one of which, hematuria, occurred in 7.4% of our sickle hemoglobinopathy children (Table 14).

TABLE 14. *INCIDENCE AND ETIOLOGY OF HEMATURIA*

A. INCIDENCE OF HEMATURIA:

	No.	*%*
Hb SS	35	8.3
Hb SC	4	5.4
Hb S-Thalassemia	2	3.5
TOTAL:	41	7.4

B. ETIOLOGY OF HEMATURIA:

	Hb SS	*Hb SC*	*Hb S-THAL.*
Related To Sickle Hemoglobin	23*	3	1
Urinary Tract Infection	7	1	1
Disseminated Intravascular Coagulopathy	5		
Acute Glomerulonephritis	2		
Platelet Dysfunction (thrombocytopathy)	1		

*2 patients had 2 and 3 episodes of hematuria for which no etiology other than Hb S could be found.

The hematuria tends to last 1 to 3 weeks and rarely requires any therapy other than bed rest and fluid replacement. In adults the problem can be more severe; lasting weeks to months and may even be life-threatening. Intravenous pyelograms on these patients generally demonstrate papillary necrosis with or without sinus tracts. In approximately one third of the children, the hematuria resulted from non-sickle related causes (glomerulonephritis, urinary tract infections, a platelet dysfunction, and disseminated intravascular coagulopathy). Therefore, all patients with hematuria need a complete renal evaluation for diagnosis and management.

ANEMIC CRISES

Both the sequestration and aplastic crises occur in 24-28% of Hb SS, 12-14% of Hb S-thalassemia, and 3-8% of Hb SC children (Table 15).

ABLE 15. *INCIDENCE OF SPLENOMEGALY, ANEMIC CRISES AND SPLENECTOMY*

NDIVIDUALS WITH:	*Hb SS*		*Hb SC*		*Hb S-THALASSEMIA*	
	No.	*%*	*No.*	*%*	*No.*	*%*
plenomegaly	229	54.5	36	48.6	18	31.6
equestration Crises	103	24.5	2	2.7	8	14.0
ther Hemolytic Episodes	22	5.2	0		0	
plenectomy For Crises	25		0		4	
plenectomy For Ruptured Spleen	0		1		0	
plastic Crises	119	28.3	6	8.1	7	12.3

Mild respiratory tract infections, usually viral in nature, have been concurrent with or have preceeded the anemic crises by 1 to 2 weeks. Live viral vaccines (measles and mumps) have precipitated 2 sequestration crises. The sequestration crisis is characterized by a sudden massive enlargement of an already enlarged spleen trapping an enormous volume of blood. Both the hemoglobin and platelet count fall, the former to levels of 1-5 gm% from the child's usual 6-9 gm% The reticulocyte count remains increased. The patients at greatest risk for sequestration crises have splenomegaly and are under 5 years of age, the majority being under 2 years of age. In our series the risk of a sequestration crisis was 44-45% for Hb SS and Hb S-thalassemia children with splenomegaly: *L.J., a 5 month old child was seen in the emergency room at 4:00 p.m. for a viral URI. Her spleen was 1 cm below the left costal margin; her hemoglobin was 8.5 gm%. Following symptomatic therapy, she returned home. At 8:00 p.m., 4 hours later, she was returned to the emergency room in shock. Her hemoglobin was 1.5 gm%; her spleen was in the left iliac fossa.*

Rapid administration of fluids and blood are necessary to prevent irreversible shock. Following the administration of whole blood or packed erythrocytes, the hemoglobin rises to levels of 2-4 gm% more than calculated from the amount of blood given. The spleen generally shrinks to the precrisis size. Since these crises tend to recur and are life-threatening, we advocate splenectomy for those patients who have a single severe crisis or who have several moderately severe crises with a markedly enlarged spleen that does not regress following transfusions. Using these criteria, 29 of our 113 patients with sequestration crises have had splenectomies. Following the splenectomy, bicillin LA 1.2 million units should be given monthly to prevent post-splenectomy infection syndrome. Prior to doing this, we had 2 children develop meningitis or sepsis, one of whom died within 4 hours of onset of her symptoms.

In contrast to the sequestration crises, aplastic crises are characterized by a more gradual decrease in hemoglobin over a 3 to 5 day period. The majority of these patients become symptomatic and seek medical assistance before their hemoglobins have fallen below 3 gm%. The reticulocyte count is less than 2% and a bone marrow generally shows maturation arrest at the basophilic or pronormoblast stage with or without a decrease in cellularity of the erythroid precursors. Occasionally in the pediatric patient with infection, a superimposed megaloblastic crisis may also be present as a result of folic acid deficiency. This occurs more frequently as the patient reaches adolescence. As a result, routine folic acid supplementation of the diet (1 to 5 mg folvite) is recommended once the child reaches puberty.

ACKNOWLEDGEMENT

I wish to express my appreciation to the many hematology fellows, technicians, nurses, clerical personnel and my close associates for their assistance in making both the clinic follow-ups and in-patient care of these patients a success. Without their assistance, we would never have accumulated the number of patients with long term follow-up that made this paper possible.

BIBLIOGRAPHY

1. Shulman, S.T., Bartlett, J., Clyde, W.A. Jr., et al: *The Unusual Severity Of Mycoplasma Pneumonia In Children With Sickle Cell Disease.* N. Engl. J. Med. 287:164-167, 1972.

2. Robinson, M.G. and Watson, R.J.: *Pneumococcal Meningitis In Sickle Cell Anemia.* N. Engl. J. of Med. 274:1006-1008, 1966.

3. Barrett-Connor, E.: *Bacterial Infection And Sickle Cell Anemia.* Medicine 50:97-112, 1971.

4. Allen, T.D.: *Pathogenesis Of Urinary Tract Infections In Children.* N. Engl. J. Med. 273:1421-1424, 1965.

5. Barrett-Connor, E.: *Infections And Sickle Cell-C Disease.* Am. J. Med. Sci. 262:162-169, 196

6. Audu, I.S.: *Sickle Cell Disease: Infections With Salmonella And Other Gram-negative Bacilli.* Paed. Indon. 4 (suppl.): 394-399, 1964.

7. Silver, H.K., Simon, J.L., and Clement, D.H.: *Salmonella Osteomyelitis And Abnormal Hemoglobin Disease.* Ped. 20:439-447, 1957.

8. Fonk, J., and Coonrod, J.D.: *Serratia Osteomyelitis In Sickle Cell Disease.* Letter to the editor, J.A.M.A. 217:80-81, 1971.

9. Rubin, H.M., Eardley, W., and Nichols, B.L.: *Shigella sonnei Osteomyelitis And Sickle Cell Anemia.* Amer. J. Dis. Chil. 116:83-87, 1968.

10. Robinson, M.G., and Halpern, C.: *Infections, Escherichia coli, And Sickle Cell Anemia.* J.A.M.A. (in press).

11. Watson, J., Burko, H., Megas, H., and Robinson,M.: *The Hand-foot Syndrome In Sickle Cell Disease In Young Children.* Pediatrics 31:975-982, 196

12. Lambotte, C.: *Hand-foot Syndrome In Sickle Cell Disease.* Letter to the editor. Am. J. Dis. of Childn. 104:200-201, 1962.

13. Greer, M., and Schotland, D.: *Abnormal Hemoglobin As A Cause Of Neurologic Disease.* Neurology 12:114-123, 1962.

14. Patterson, R.H., Wilson, H., and Diggs, L.W.: *Sickle Cell Anemia: A Surgical Problem II.* Surgery 28:393-403, 1950.

UNSOLVED MYSTERIES IN GENETIC COUNSELING

Robert F. Murray, Jr., M.D.

INTRODUCTION

There are a number of unsolved mysteries in sickle cell disease. Among them is the mystery of the contact points responsible for the structure of sickle cell hemoglobin microtubules. There is the mystery of small vessel disease that leads to the pain and tissue damage that occurs in sickle cell crisis. There is the mystery of the milder forms of sickle cell disease that have been found in increasing numbers of patients and there are unsolved mysteries in the process of genetic counseling. Not only are there areas of ignorance about genetic counseling, but there is still some dispute about what name to give this essential adjunct to sickle cell testing. It probably isn't very important whether we call the process genetic counseling, biomedical counseling or educational counseling. What is important is what takes place during the process of counseling and how to make the process as effective as possible. For the sake of this discussion, the term "genetic counseling" will be used because it is the one that is best known.

THE MYSTERIOUS PROCESS OF GENETIC COUNSELING

If the process of genetic counseling is dissected, we can see that there are at least four key points that must be addressed. It is important to know what is meant by counseling, what the counselor hopes counseling will accomplish, what the counselee expects to happen, and what happens as a result of counseling.

Genetic counseling has operated under many definitions [1,2,3] but in the context of modern medical practice and its concern with the whole patient a more comprehensive definition of genetic counseling is in order. In this context genetic counseling can be defined as the process of communicating all the factors that relate to the disease or condition in question including the manifestations of the disease, the prognosis of the disease, the genetics of the disease and the alternatives of one or another course of action. It cannot be over emphasized that the total picture of the condition rather than only parts of it must be dealt with. This is especially important because so many individuals have no real concept of what a person with sickle cell disease or one of the other hemoglobinopathies is really like. They merely picture a person who suffers from pain or who is in misery or who is deformed and so it is important that this distorted concept be altered. There will be occasional situations when the counselee is an individual who has one of the sickle cell diseases in mild form. It is essential that they have a clear understanding of what the possible consequences of having the disease might be so that they will take seriously the need for careful monitoring of their condition by the physicians. On the other hand, a balanced picture of the prognosis for sickle cell disease must be presented. Not only must they be aware of the serious nature of the disease, but also the fact that with good medical care they can avoid or postpone some of the complications of the disease and improve their chance of living active and productive lives. This is especially difficult when the person with the sickle cell disease has only mild anemia and has never had any clinical symptoms that incapacitated them. In some cases, the patients resist accepting the information that they do have an illness. By ignoring the advice of the counselor such an individual may place themselves in positions that could be disastrous for their physical well-being.

Communication is at the heart of the counseling process. This is true of any interaction between two or more human beings, but it is here where one of the perplexing mysteries of genetic counseling is found. For there is only the vaguest notion about how much information is transmitted from counselor to counselee.

It also isn't clear how much of the information the counselee understands.

Much experience and many studies have shown that the more feedback there is between two communicating individuals the more likely is the information to be correctly transmitted, correctly received and understood. This is also assumed to be true in genetic counseling. More often than not in the medical setting the bulk of communication flows from the counselor or physician to the counselee. In an effective counseling situation, there must be an increased feedback from the counselee in the form of questions or comments which should be encouraged by the counselor (see figure 1).

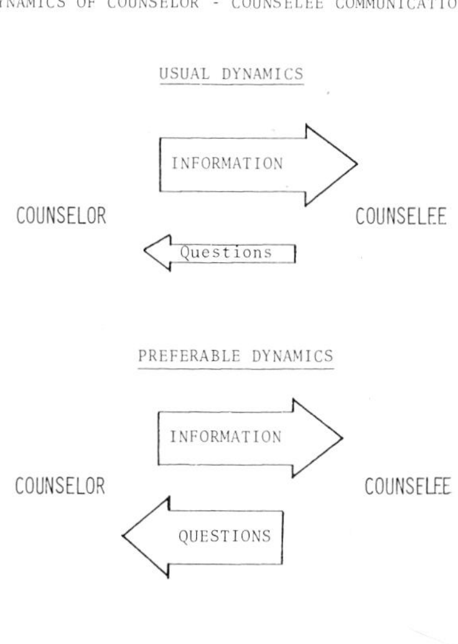

Fig. 1. This illustrates in simplified form the dynamics of communication between counselor and counselee that are found in the usual counseling situation (above) and preferable situation (below). A greater flow of questions from counselee to counselor should be encouraged since this almost always improves communication.

It is probably true that the success of communication in the counseling session is directly proportional to the number of questions asked and comments made by the counselee. One excellent way of beginning the counseling session in a manner that will encourage communication is for the counselor to make the following statement: *"Please feel free to ask any question at all that comes to mind. There is no such thing as a silly question. This time is yours and must be used to your best advantage."* If the counselee really believes this statement, he or she will not be reluctant to ask questions about words or phrases that are unfamiliar to them.

A second mystery surrounding the counseling process is a consequence of the factors which influence the interaction between counselor and counselee. One major factor is the effect of motivation of counselor and counselee. There can be little doubt that the counselee who has sought genetic counseling and is prepared to receive the information about sickle cell disease is going to be much more receptive and aware than the counselee who has been sought out by the counselor and given information without the proper mental set as in some screening programs that are going on around the country. On the other hand, it has been argued that it is better to have a little information poorly understood than no information at all. The mystery of counselee motivation in genetic counseling needs much closer study. Another important factor in the counseling process is the educational background of counselor as well as counselee. Preliminary studies from the genetic counseling program associated with the Howard University Center for Sickle Cell Anemia has provided preliminary data consistent with this fact. Studies of information transfer show that there is a positive correlation between educational background and the amount of information which is received and understood. A third point of importance relates to the emotional background of counselor and counselee. One assumes that the emotional state of the counselor is generally positive and stable. However, it is possible that on a given day or during a given period the counselor may be emotionally upset or not be focused on the task of counseling. During these periods, counselors should excuse themselves from doing any counseling since their feelings are readily transmitted to the counselees and will interfere. In the vast majority of cases, counselees are anxious and sometimes depressed by the knowledge that they either carry the sickle cell gene or have a sickle cell disease. One of the essential aspects of the counseling process is to relieve the anxiety of counselees or to detect depression so that it can be dealt with in a positive and constructive fashion. It is well known that there is an important psychiatric component involved in communication between individuals and when anxiety predominates, effective communication is interfered with.

If counseling has been successful, then the following should hold:

1. *The counselees have received the information.*
2. *They have understood the information.*
3. *The counselee can make his or her own decision which is in their best interest.*

It cannot be over emphasized that the decisions of the counselees are those which meet their needs rather than the needs of medicine or mankind in general. In other words, it is reasonable for some couples where both carry sickle cell trait to choose to take the 25% risk of having a child with sickle cell disease. Even though we may feel as physicians the risk is too high, this should not be transmitted as the proper decision for the counselees to make. Even if the counselee makes no decision (which in itself is a decision of sorts) one cannot say that the counseling has been a waste of time. After all, a great deal of what we do in medicine is to provide the individual with information through which they may make decisions about what to do with their own life situation.

The counseling process itself can be divided into four rather distinctive phases. These can be listed as follows:

1. *The phase of counselee characterization.*
2. *The phase of counselee education.*
3. *An evaluative phase.*
4. *The phase of follow-up.*

These phases are of course not clearly distinctive or necessarily easily distinguished one from another. Some of the phases such as education and characterization may go on simultaneously. Evaluation can occur in the initial counseling session as well as in follow-up counseling sessions.

Counselees should be characterized at least with respect to the following variables:

1. *What misconceptions do they have about sickle cell disease?*
2. *Do they have any medical complaints or problems which they think may be caused by sickle cell trait?*
3. *Is there a family history of sickle cell disease?*
4. *Do they have specific questions on their minds?*

There are, of course, other points of characterization which can be considered. In order to be certain that all counselees are characterized in the same way, we use a standard form to collect at least a minimal amount of information on each one. This baseline of information is essential in future evaluations of the effectiveness of the counseling program.

During the second or educational phase of counseling, basic information must be transmitted to; *1.) correct prior misconceptions* and *2.) provide the counselee with baseline information that will permit them to understand sickle cell disease, the genetics thereof and make decisions appropriate to their own life situation.* This constitutes one of the major goals of the counseling process and must be carried out carefully, thoughtfully and thoroughly. It is one of the few aspects of counseling that can be reasonably and accurately evaluated, on one sense, through written questionnaires.[4]

The effectiveness of a counseling program can only be determined by evaluation. Evaluation is a rather complex process when done properly and thoroughly.[5] However, it is possible, by less complex means, to determine the effectiveness of the educational aspect of counseling. It is also possible, but with somewhat greater difficulty, to evaluate the psychological and emotional aspects of the counseling process. The educational aspect of counseling can be evaluated in three ways; *1.) by use of a simple diagram which the counselee uses to illustrate their understanding of recurrence risks after the genetics of the process have been explained; 2.) by asking questions of the counselee, frequently to determine whether they understand what they are being told; 3.) by having them complete a short answer multiple choice questionnaire based upon key points of information that have been transmitted to the counselees during the counseling process.* This type of evaluation can be carried out immediately after counseling at some time during follow-up counseling or at some months after the counseling process has been completed. In order to evaluate in a more long-range fashion the retention of information in counseling, we have chosen to mail a multiple choice questionnaire to counselees approximately 2 months after they have been counseled, ask them to complete the questionnaire and return it to us in a stamped, self-addressed envelope. Approximately half of the counselees returned these questionnaires for evaluation enabling us to get some idea of the effectiveness of the educational process.

Evaluation of the emotional aspects of the counseling process is performed by asking the counselees what their reactions to counseling have been or by noting their behavior and response to counseling in some standard fashion. It is essential that the counselor indicate in his or her record of the counseling session their subjective evaluation of the counseling process. Follow-up has been found to be an absolutely essential element in all programs dealing with health care. Genetic counseling for the hemoglobinopathies is no exception to this rule. Not only because the initial counseling session may be highly emotionally charged, but also because counselees may be unfamiliar with medical and genetic concepts, additional reinforcement of information transmitted as well as correction of misconceptions should be carried out during one or more subsequent counseling sessions. Not only that, it is important to maintain contact with counselees so that other members of the family who are at risk to be carriers of genes determining sickle cell hemoglobinopathies and who therefore should be tested and counseled, can be reached and brought in for testing. Follow-up is especially vital when one is working with couples who are at risk to give birth to children with sickle cell disease. Such couples go through a prolonged period of agonizing over decisions which they might wish to make and it is not unusual for them to change their minds several times in the course of one or two years. The counselor should be ready to discuss and rediscuss the educational aspects of the counseling process as many times as necessary and to provide emotional and medical support when necessary. It is still not apparent what the long-range effects of these efforts will be.

Although these phases of the counseling process appear to be clearly delineated, it is probable that this is only a minimum subdivision of a complex process which is heavily and emotionally loaded. It has been suggested by some counselors that all persons involved in genetic counseling should have a strong psychiatric, psychological background in order to be able to deal in the most sensitive way possible with the variety of medical and emotional problems that may be presented by counselees who initially come for genetical counseling in the hemoglobinopathies.

EDUCATIONAL MATERIALS AND METHODS IN COUNSELING

Communication of scientific information to the laymen or to individuals unfamiliar with medical terminolog is a difficult task at best. There is the problem of heterogeneity of educational background, motivation, and intellectual ability. Add to this the relative skill of different counselors and one has an extremely difficult situation to evaluate and the complexity of trying to educate an individual about a complex medical topic in a few relatively brief contacts is obvious. Health educators have been studying this process for many years and genetic counselors have been involved in it for a relatively brief period of time. To indicate that anyone knows the best way to do this is, of course, ridiculous. There is much to learn and probably many different ways to communicate the basic information and facts about sickle cell anemia and sickle cell trait. We have struggled with this problem for several years at our center and have developed a set of approximately 20 or so slides which are used with a twin viewer so that comparisons are permitted. That is to say, it is possible to show normal and abnormal conditions side-by-side simultaneously so that the counselee can make comparisons for themselves. Other centers have also developed audiovisual materials which in some ways are suitable and in some ways, in our judgement, perhaps not. We do feel that it is important to illustrate certain basic concepts and the slides we have developed, at least, and begin to do this. One must maintain a very flexible attitude about educational materials and should try from time to time different variations of illustrations and presentations in order to improve the presentations that are made. Ideally, one would like to have controlled studies that would illustrate which materials are most effective in communicating information to individuals of a given average educational background.

The following is a list of the slides which are used in counseling and the points they are meant to illustrate. The precise appearance of the slides is not critical. Rather, the information to be illustrated and the concepts being presented are most important and should be emphasized. It is important for individuals to prepare their own visual materials based upon this format or those at other centers using their own imagination to improve upon the format that is presented. One cannot over emphasize the importance of being certain that the basic point to be communicated is clearly understood by the counselee before proceeding to the next point:

Slide 1. *This slide shows the basic shape of the normal human red blood cell.*

Slide 2. *This slide illustrates the shape and flexibility of the normal red blood cell.*

Slide 3. *This slide illustrates the variety of shapes and forms of the sickled red blood cell.*

Slide 4. This slide illustrates the linear and rod-like arrangement of the hemoglobin within sickle cells that causes the cell to take the sickled shape when oxygen is removed.

Slide 5. This slide illustrates the mechanism by which hemoglobin molecules stick to one another to form the long rods of hemoglobin that distort the red blood cell.

Slide 6. This slide shows the branching and progressive narrowing of the circulatory system in order to illustrate the places where sickle cells get trapped and block the circulation. It also shows why sickle cells have a shape that causes sludging of blood flow. The counselee will better understand the problems of circulation and what a capillary is like.

Slide 7. This slide illustrates the concept of amino acids as building blocks of the protein and the manner in which a change in the gene produces a change in the amino acid or building block unit. It shows the change from glutamic acid to valine in the case of sickle cell anemia and lysine in the case of hemoglobin C.

Slide 8. This slide shows the changed appearance in an African child produced by moderate to severe sickle cell anemia. The shape of the head, the thin arms and legs, and the swollen belly should be noted.

Slide 9. This slide shows two brothers who have a milder form of sickle cell anemia and who appear essentially healthy.

Slide 10. This slide illustrates in simplified form the sequence of changes that produce the clinical symptoms of sickle cell anemia.

Slide 11. This slide illustrates the essential combinations of genes in egg and sperm that produce children with sickle cell anemia and sickle cell trait.

Slide 12a. This slide illustrates the possible kinds of offspring when 2 parents with sickle cell trait have children.

Slide 12b. This slide illustrates the possible kinds of offspring when one parent with sickle cell anemia and one parent with sickle cell trait have children.

Slide 12c. This slide illustrates the possible kinds of offspring when one parent with sickle cell trait and one parent with hemoglobin C trait have children.

Slide 13a. *This side shows a simplified illustration of the genetic make-up of children when one parent has sickle cell trait and one parent carried the usual hemoglobin.*
Slide 13b. *This slide illustrates the genetic make-up of children when both parents have sickle cell trait.*
Slide 14. *This slide illustrates the distribution of the sickle cell gene in the eastern hemisphere.*
Slide 15. *This slide illustrates the distribution of falciparum malaria in the eastern hemisphere.*
Slide 16. *This slide shows common genetically determined conditions in areas of the world where they are found and consequently the types of people who will be affected by them.*
Slide 17. *This slide shows the results of the dithionite or Sickledex* R *test.*
Slide 18. *This slide illustrates the appearance of different hemoglobin types on cellulose acetate electrophoresis.*

THE MYSTERY OF RECURRENCE RISK

The difficulty of illustrating the recurrence risk in genetic counseling should not be under emphasized. This is because a true understanding of the statistical aspect of recurrence risk is one which is most frequently understood by the counselees. For this reason, we spend a great deal of time demonstrating how the union of sperm carrying sickle cell gene with egg carrying sickle cell gene is essential for the inheritance of sickle cell anemia. Figure 2 is an illustration used in our counseling session to make the point that both parents must carry the sickle cell gene in order for a child to inherit sickle cell anemia or that each parent must carry an abnormal hemoglobinopathy gene in order for a child to inherit sickle cell anemia or sickle cell disease. Figure 3 illustrates the 1 in 4 recurrence risk in the form of a Punnett square which again emphasizes the fact that the genetic make-up of the child relative to the hemoglobinopathies is based on the genes in the egg and sperm of the parent rather than on how many children have occurred in the family. Although other methods of illustrating this are used, we feel that this method helps the counselee to a clearer understanding of the recurrence risk. That is, that the recurrence risk stays the same for each child born.

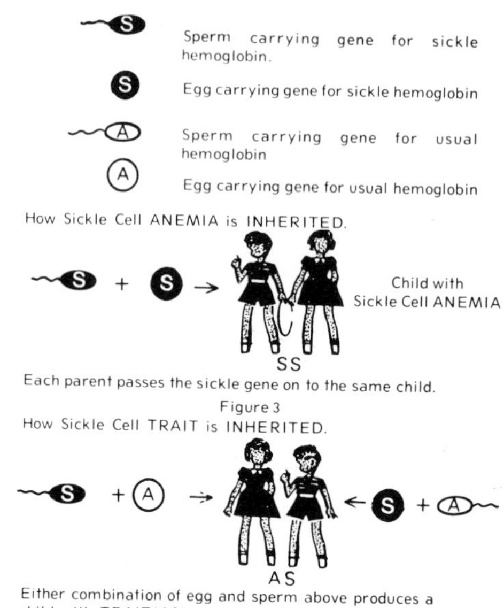

Fig. 2. This shows the types of hemoglobin genes that are carried by egg and sperm when a child with sickle cell anemia is produced (above) and when a child with sickle cell trait is produced.

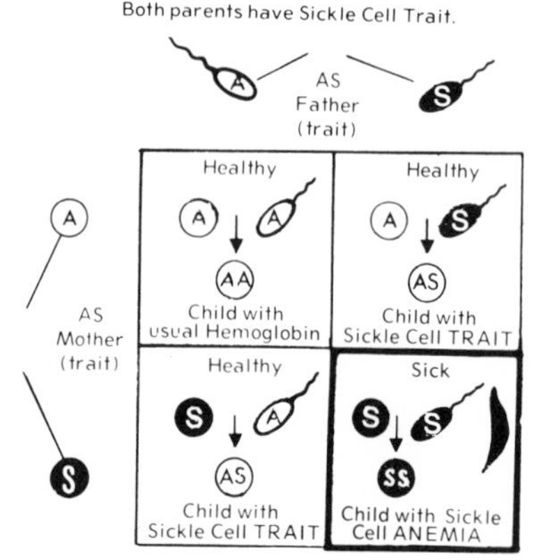

Fig. 3. This diagram shows how the 1 in 4 or 25% recurrence risk of having a child with sickle cell anemia (SS) results from the mating of two people with sickle cell trait (AS).

Figure 4 shows this recurrence risk when one parent has sickle cell anemia and one carries sickle cell trait. It emphasizes the increase in recurrence risk.

One parent has Sickle Cell Trait

One parent has Sickle Cell Anemia

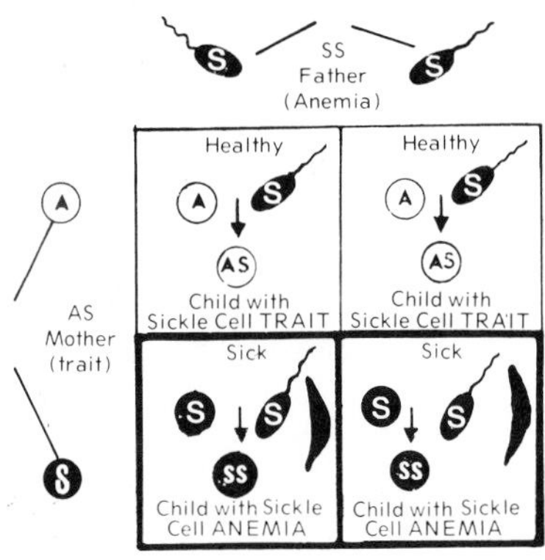

2 out of 4 (50%) chance of having a child with Sickle Cell Anemia.

Fig. 4. This diagram shows how the 1 in 2 or 50% recurrence risk of having a child with sickle cell anemia (SS) results from the mating of one person with sickle cell anemia (SS) and one person with sickle cell trait (AS).

At this point, we go to the mini-test which is shown in Figure 6 and ask the counselee to give us the recurrence risk for a child with sickle cell anemia if one parent had sickle cell anemia and the other does not have the trait or the anemia or any abnormal hemoglobinopathy gene. Seven out of 10 individuals answer correctly that the recurrence risk is 0 and realize immediately that all children would have sickle cell trait. Figure 5 illustrates how having a different hemoglobinopathy gene, namely hemoglobin C, can produce the same 1 in 4 or 25% recurrence risk for having an affected child if each child is a carrier.

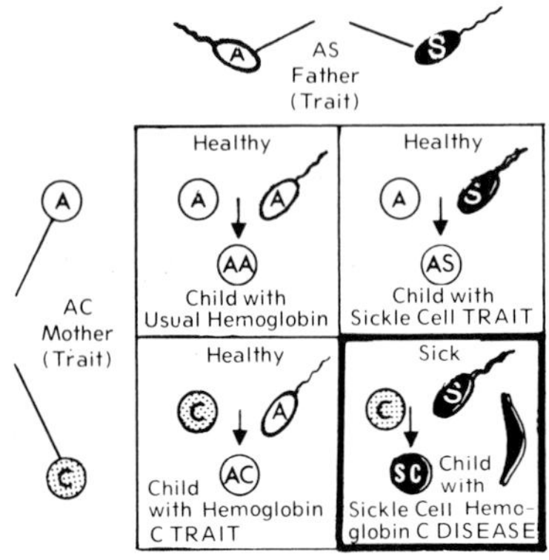

Fig. 5. This diagram shows how the 1 in 4 or 25% recurrence risk of having a child with sickle cell hemoglobin C disease (SC) results from the mating of one person with sickle cell trait (AS) and one person with hemoglobin C trait (AC).

There are, of course, other ways of illustrating this recurrence risk, but we feel that our experience has taught us that patients can figure this out for themselves once they can break down the translation of the genetic status of the parent into the genetic status of eggs and sperm. Another way of illustrating this point is to use dice which are color coded. A die representing sickle cell trait will have 3 sides colored in one way and 3 in another to illustrate that half of the eggs or sperm will carry the sickled gene and half will not. Two such die can then be thrown repeatedly by the counselee to show how it is not possible to predict ahead of time what the child will be even though the odds for having a child that does not have sickle cell trait is 3 out of 4 or 75%. One can also use paper plates which have been cut in half and colored with different colors. One-half will represent the sickle cell gene and the

MINI-TESTS FOR THE COUNSELEE

Fill in the squares to represent the offspring of the matings shown below:

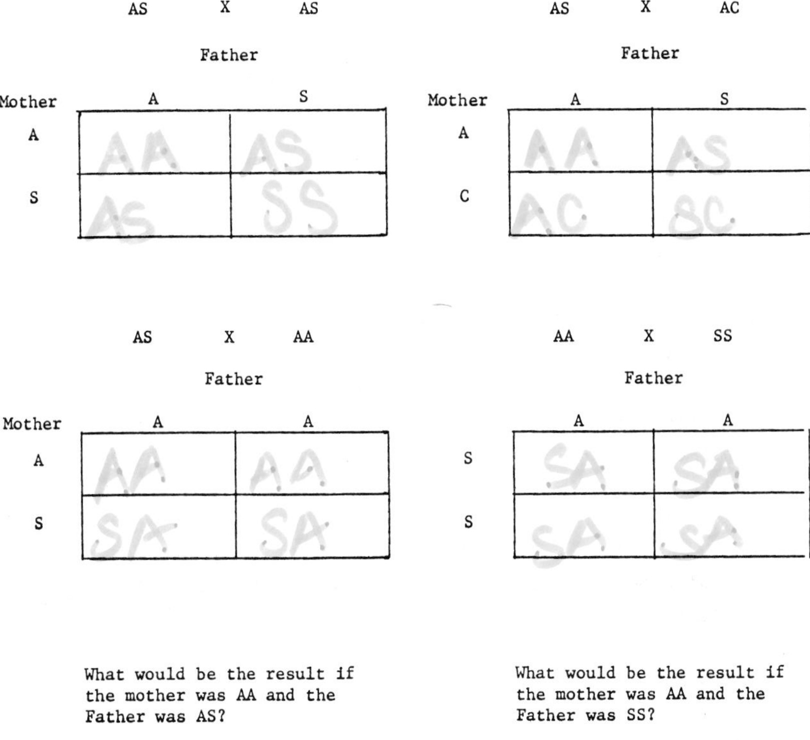

Fig. 6. Mini-test that can be used during counseling session to determine whether counselee understands the derivation of genetic recurrence risk.

other the usual gene for hemoglobin A. Each member of a couple or the counselor or counselee may at random take from behind their backs one of these halves as if they were simulating the union of egg and sperm. One can do this over and over again to illustrate the point that the recurrence risk cannot be predicted in advance. Finally, one could develop a kind of color-coded wheel which can be spun by the counselee in the fashion of a roulette wheel to illustrate the fact that it is not possible to predict the recurrence risk in advance. The whole idea is to make clear to the counselee that the union of the 2 sickle cell genes is a chance phenomenon over which we have, at the moment, no control. For unknown reasons even people who are experienced gamblers have difficulty understanding the concept of recurrence risk. It is a real mystery why someone who understands the odds on a racing form is confused by the 1 in 4 risk in sickle cell disease. Perhaps when we understand this mystery we can do a better job explaining the odds.

THE PROBLEM OF NON-PATERNITY AND MUTATION

It is important to spend some time illustrating the origin of the gene. It should be stressed that all mutations occur at all times, in all racial and ethnic groups that the sickle cell mutation continues to occur, but that the environment in all places where malaria is an endemic disease does not favor the increase in its frequency. A small number of white individuals who do not have Greek or Italian ancestry will be found to have sickle cell trait for this reason.

Another point which does not get emphasized, but which should be, is the fact that nonpaternity can be detected when sickle cell testing is carried out. This is a very delicate and serious matter which is difficult to handle and which requires an enormous amount of sensitivity to deal without causing a break-up in the family. One can handle this problem in several ways, but there are two ways which we use to avoid arousing undue suspicion in families where there is stability and love. *1.) We emphasize strongly that the occurence of genetic discrepancy, that is, the situation where both parents do not have sickle cell trait and a child has sickle cell trait is a result of gene mutation. If parents press the issue, we may then go into the possibility of laboratory error or a clerical error and request a repeat study. If a repeat study is done, it is possible to then "label" one of the parents, usually the mother, as having sickle cell trait. One cannot emphasize too strongly that it is important to repeat such tests in order to be certain that the results are accurate and that there has not been clerical error. 2.) We may provide the explanation given above and then request a conference with the mother privately in order to raise the question of nonpaternity with her. Not infrequently the mother does state that there is the possibility that the child is not the result of the union between her and the current father. In this case, it is explained to her that if she has no further children with anyone but the legal father, she will not have any further children with sickle cell trait and the situation will not occur again.*

Of course, the ethical and moral issues surrounding withholding information and the possibility that this information could come out later leaves a certain element of risk here. On the other hand, in our society today the stigma attached to children born out of wedlock or the trauma to the ego of a male who has raised children that are not his, can be terribly strong and lead to the break-up of an otherwise happy family. There is, of course, no easy answer to this question and the counselor should have a good understanding of the family constellation and the stresses and strain they may be experiencing before he or she attempts to deal with this problem.

Because the frequency of nonpaternity even in so-called "good middle class families" is 5-7% and is probably higher in inner-city Black communities, it must be considered as a significant factor when genetic counseling is to be provided in large-scale screening operations. It is not a problem to be ignored. If one assumes that the frequency of nonpaternity is 7%, (it is probably closer to 10-15% in some inner-city communities) the chance of detecting nonpaternity in a screening program is 1 in every 250 couples screened. This means that in a large-scale screening situation in which 10,000 individuals or 5,000 couples might be screened, one may detect approximately 20 examples of nonpaternity. This is one situation in which the team approach or multidisciplinary approach to counseling cannot be overstressed. The combined efforts of a sensitive social worker, perhaps a psychiatrist and the counselor including the primary physician may be required to handle a rather delicate situation.

OPTIONS FOR COUPLES AT RISK: THE MYSTERY OF DECISION-MAKING

A review of the reproductive options for couples at risk should not be undertaken until it is clear that the couple involved understands all the background information, and the psychodynamics of the situation are well understood. At this point, the reproductive options for couples at risk may be reviewed. These include: *1.) that the couple take the 25% recurrence risk because the desire for children is still great; 2.) that they abstain from childbearing until there is better treatment for sickle cell anemia; 3.) that they abstain from childbearing and adopt children; 4.) that one have artificial insemination of the wife by a donor who does not have sickle cell trait; 5.) that there is artificial insemination of a surrogate mother who does not have sickle cell trait using sperm taken from the husband of the couple.*

A combination of the latter two options will allow each parent at this point in time to have a child that is biologically half theirs and not undergo the risk of having a child with sickle cell disease. Option number 3 is more and more difficult because of the greater shortage of adoptable children. The hope, of course, is that some effective treatment of sickle cell anemia will be found so that parents can take the risk and the emphasis will then be on early detection of potentially affected children through newborn screening. Considerable work is going on to determine the means of identifying affected children in the first trimester of pregnancy so that therapeutic abortion might be offered.

However, the ethical and moral conflict surrounding the fact that an individual with sickle cell anemia need not be severely affected, but may live a reasonably productive and active life as an individual, raises some serious moral questions about this as a recommended means of dealing with sickle cell anemia. It is true, however, that many couples will choose this option if it were currently available. It should also be stated that no one center has studied enough couples to know what their choice would be with regard to the reproductive options that are listed. It cannot be over emphasized, however, that the couple should make their own decision. The decision should not be that of the counselor or physician. One should not under emphasize the fact that many couples at risk are fortunate not to have any affected children at all and that the majority of couples, if they have 3 children will have only one affected child by chance.

The decisions that couples faced with this dilemma will make it still a great mystery. One cannot necessarily extrapolate from the decision made by couples at risk to have children with other kinds of genetic disease since there is some evidence suggesting that the burden of the disease, as perceived by the parents, is a much more significant factor in the decision that parents make about recurrence risks than the recurrence risk itself.

EFFECTIVENESS OF INFORMATION TRANSFER IN COUNSELING

We have been counseling for sickle cell anemia and sickle cell trait for several years now and have been evaluating our counseling experience for the last 2 years. By having a uniform set of counselors, all of whom are physicians trained in medical genetics and the counseling techniques, and following up with a 20 question questionnaire dealing with the main points delivered in the counseling session, we have found that based on a sample of approximately a third of the individuals counseled, the majority of individuals retained 70% or more of the information transmitted to them. That despite our efforts, most of them still have difficulty with understanding statistical recurrence risks. Finally, it is clear that the retention of information is correlated with marital status and level of education. It is also apparent that the counseling session which is not good or excellent should clearly be repeated in detail since information transfer as measured by our test is not adequate in such sessions. We must find better ways of communicating the basic information in sickle cell disease and, in addition, find ways of communicating more effectively to individuals whose educational level is low or whose motivation is poor.

GENETIC COUNSELING, AN EVOLVING DISCIPLINE

Genetic counseling is still evolving. We are learning more about the communications process, the ways of communicating and the psychodynamics involved in the process. In the final analysis, the most effective counseling will be carried out in individuals who have been well educated in advance and where we will deal not with the basic information involved, but with the personal problems which the individuals themselves experienced in either understanding the basic information or in translating it into meaning in their personal lives.

We must do a very long-term study of what individuals do with counseling information because we still don't know whether or not it has any effect on the decisions that they make in terms of reproduction or their lives in general. Only by doing such a study, probably on a large-scale, collaborative basis with centers across the country we will be able to do the best job of counseling for the counselees and have a significant impact on the problem of management of sickle cell anemia and other sickle cell diseases. The question of who should do the counseling is a difficult one, but it is clear that in different situations different individuals are better suited to provide counseling. If we have "a counseling team" to relate to the wide variety of patien who have different problems, we would perhaps be able to do the best job rather than arguing the very controversial issue as to whether M.D.'s, Ph.D.'s or social worke should be the primary counselors. We must remember that the counselees are most important in this process and all we do should be for their benefit.

REFERENCES

1. Fraser, F.C.: *Counseling in Genetics: Its Intent and Scope.* In Birth Defects Orig. Art. Ser., ed. D. Bergsma, *Genetic Counseling.* Published by Williams and Wilkins Co., Baltimore, M.D. for the National Foundation, March of Dimes, White Plains, N.Y., VI (1):7, 1970.

2. Sly, W.S.: *What is Genetic Counseling?* In Birth Defects Orig. Art. Ser., ed. D. Bergsma, in *Contemporary Genetic Counseling.* Published by the National Foundation, March of Dimes, White Plains, N.Y., IX (4):5, 1973.

3. Kallman, F.J.: *Some Aspects of Genetic Counseling.* In Neel, J.V., Shaw, I.W., and Schull, W.J. (ed.). *Genetics and the Epidemiology of Chronic Diseases.* U.S. Department of Health, Education and Welfare, 1965.

4. Deniston, O.L., Rosenstock, I.M. and Getting, V.A.: *Evaluation of Program Effectiveness.* Public Health Reports 83:323-336, 1968.

5. Deniston, O.L., Rosenstock, I.M., Welch, W. and Getting, V.A.: *Evaluation of Program Efficiency.* Public Health Reports 83:603-610, 1968.

SUBJECT INDEX